VACCINE

VACCINE

The Debate in Modern America

MARK A. LARGENT

The Johns Hopkins University Press

Baltimore

© 2012 The Johns Hopkins University Press
All rights reserved. Published 2012
Printed in the United States of America on acid-free paper
9 8 7 6 5 4 3 2 1

The Johns Hopkins University Press
2715 North Charles Street
Baltimore, Maryland 21218-4363
www.press.jhu.edu

Library of Congress Cataloging-in-Publication Data
Largent, Mark A.
     Vaccine : the debate in modern America / Mark A. Largent.
        p. ; cm.
     Includes bibliographical references and index.
     ISBN 978-1-4214-0607-7 (hdbk. : alk. paper) — ISBN 1-4214-0607-1
(hdbk. : alk. paper) — ISBN 978-1-4214-0672-5 (electronic) — ISBN
1-4214-0672-1 (electronic)
     I. Title.
     [DNLM: 1. Vaccines—adverse effects—United States.   2. Attitude to
Health—United States.   3. Autistic Disorder—etiology—United States.
4. Dissent and Disputes—United States. QW 805]
615.3'72—dc23   2011048241

A catalog record for this book is available from the British Library.

*Special discounts are available for bulk purchases of this book. For
more information, please contact Special Sales at 410-516-6936 or
specialsales@press.jhu.edu.*

The Johns Hopkins University Press uses environmentally friendly
book materials, including recycled text paper that is composed of at least
30 percent post-consumer waste, whenever possible.

To my friend,
Chris Young

Thank you, Chris, for all of your support,
encouragement, and guidance

CONTENTS

VACCINE

Introduction

Over the past decade, American parents have become increasingly anxious about following their pediatricians' recommendations to fully vaccinate their children. As a result, about 40 percent of American parents today have chosen to delay certain vaccines or outright refuse to allow their children's physicians to vaccinate their children with one or more of the recommended or mandated vaccines. Their anxieties arise from several sources, but the most widely discussed concern among parents is the claim that vaccines may cause autism. Despite assurances from every mainstream scientific and medical institution that vaccines do not cause autism, millions of parents fear that they do, and it shapes their decisions about whether and when to vaccinate their children.[1]

The modern American debate over vaccines and autism is a proxy debate. It is a debate in which both sides uphold claims that are simplistic stand-ins for real problems. Underlying parents' fears about a link between vaccines and autism are a complex set of concerns about the modern vaccine schedule that they rarely articulate clearly. Health officials prefer to debate within the limited terms of the claim that vaccines cause autism, because it frames the debate in terms that are familiar to them and because the autism question keeps the controversy within the confines of their scientific and technical expertise. It also allows health officials to avoid admitting that many of the concerns of parents are not scientific in nature, and thus scientists and physicians can have only a limited say in alleviating them.

This book is an account of the emergence of the modern American vaccine controversy. It reveals that, while the polemicists have debated within the confines of the vaccines-cause-autism argument, serious real problems with the current vaccine regime remain unresolved. These problems are discussed in detail in the book's final chapter. For now, it is enough to say that the debate about vaccines and autism obscures serious problems—some inherent to the vaccines themselves and some unintentionally generated over the last several decades—that animate parents' anxieties about vaccines. The entire process is conducted under substantial time and financial pressures; so many shots are given at such a young age against so many obscure diseases without parents' having a clear understanding of why we are vaccinating against certain diseases and not others. No reasonable person ought to be surprised that the process has created apprehension among thoughtful parents.

This is not a history of bogeymen conjured by parents who simply distrust modern science, nor is it a story of how scientists and physicians have silenced quacks. It is a description of how, lacking a clear long-term vision, we have drifted into a situation in which vaccines, one of the most effective tools in the public health arsenal, have become the source of tremendous angst among the very people charged with the power to allow pediatricians to vaccinate children against deadly and debilitating ailments. As we continue to add more and more new vaccines to the already long list of recommended and mandated vaccines, we are priming ourselves for a breakdown of parents' trust in vaccines and in mainstream medicine generally.

For Her Own Good

My interest in the modern American vaccine debate emerged on April 6, 2006, when my first child, Annabelle, was born. That same day, *USA Today* published an advertisement claiming that the 6,000 percent increase in autism that Americans had witnessed during the 1990s was the result of the "ambitious immunization schedule" that the Centers for Disease Control and Prevention (CDC) had adopted. The advertisement claimed that the CDC had more than tripled the number of vaccines required for children before they started kindergarten. Several parent groups, each of which focused in some way on the relationship between vaccines and autism, sponsored the advertisement. They demanded the complete elimination of mercury from all vaccines and a reevaluation of the combined effects of the nearly three dozen mandated and recommended vaccines that children received by the time they were six years old.[2]

A few hours after her first breath, Annabelle received her first vaccination, half a milliliter of Merck's Recombivax HB, which promised to prevent her from contracting hepatitis B. The nurse explained that Annabelle would either get the shot that day or she would get it three days later, when we took her to her first pediatrician appointment. The benefit of getting it now, she said, was to avoid the $15 insurance copayment that the pediatrician would have to collect. "Either way," the nurse told us, "she has to get the vaccine, because it is the law." Michigan state law does indeed mandate the hepatitis B vaccine—along with vaccines for ten other communicable diseases—for all children who attend childcare centers, preschools, and schools.[3]

Months later, as I grew increasingly interested in the ongoing public controversy over vaccines, I learned that in fact we did not have to give our daughter a required vaccine to send her to daycare or later to public school because "mandated" in this context does not mean that she must get the vaccine. It turns out that in Michigan, as in many other states, health authorities have little power to coerce us into vaccinating our children. I also later learned that, motivated by a $15 savings, my wife and I had agreed to allow the nurse to vaccinate our day-old daughter against a disease that she could probably only contract by having sex with an infected person or by sharing contaminated needles with an infected drug addict. Why would the state require us to vaccinate Annabelle against hepatitis B given that it would take years—or, better, decades—before she had any risk of contracting the disease?[4]

Every state has a list of vaccines that it compels all children to receive. Generally, the most effective method of getting parents to vaccinate their children is to require that they present up-to-date immunization records to daycare and school officials before their children can attend public schools or licensed daycare facilities. All states allow parents to secure from their children's doctors an exemption from any particular vaccine for medical reasons, such as compromised immune systems or allergies, but only about 1 percent of all U.S. children have such exceptions. Every state except Mississippi and West Virginia also allows children to be exempted from vaccination for religious reasons, the details of which vary from state to state and can include specific religious sects' restrictions against vaccinations, refusal to vaccinate because some vaccines were prepared using cell lines that may have been derived from aborted fetuses, and in some states for religious beliefs against injecting foreign substances into one's body. As with medical exemptions, the percentage of children with religious exemptions to mandated vaccines is relatively low, usually no more than 2 percent in any particular state.

In recent years, a third category of exemption has emerged, the philosophical or personal belief exemption. It varies from state to state and can include justifications drawn from parents' political, ideological, or religious views, their chosen lifestyles, and even their personal opinions or political beliefs. Often, parents only have to sign a form stating they have a philosophical objection to vaccination, and at most they need to appear in person or present a signed and notarized form claiming their objection. In many states, obtaining an exemption requires much less effort from the parent than does fulfilling immunization requirements. This was indeed the case for me recently. Annabelle's daycare notified me that she had not yet received a mandated vaccine, and I was unable to get an appointment with her pediatrician quickly enough to satisfy the daycare's requirements. So, I simply filled out an exemption form and wrote "philosophically opposed to mandatory vaccinations" in the area labeled "Reasons." A couple of months later, after I was able to get her into the pediatrician's office, I handed the daycare's administrative assistant an updated vaccination record and Annabelle was no longer among the children with a philosophical exemption.[5]

By 2006, twenty states allowed for philosophical exemptions, some of the nation's most populous states among them. More than half of U.S. parents now have the option to exempt their children from mandated vaccines on the basis of philosophical objections. Over the last several years, public health authorities have become increasingly concerned about the effects of these easily obtained exemptions in reducing "vaccine compliance rates," the formal term for the percentage of children who have received all their mandated shots. A 2001 study of the processes for obtaining an exemption for mandated vaccinations found that states with the easiest requirements for exemption also had the highest percentage of them. The growing number of available exemptions and their increasing use by parents highlight the fact that, in the United States, vaccinating our children is a parent's choice, and increasingly parents are recognizing their rights to choose for or against particular vaccines or vaccines generally.[6]

At almost every "well-baby" doctor visit during her first two years, Annabelle received at least one of her mandated vaccines. Because a sick child cannot be vaccinated, the periodic well-baby visits are the only time outside of specific trips to the doctor's office that she could get the nearly three dozen shots that she is expected to receive before she starts kindergarten. Anyone who has pinned down their child for a shot—or in some cases three or four shots administered quickly one after another—knows the trauma both parents and children experience as well as the mantra parents repeat in their minds as their kids scream in pain, fear, and frustration: "This is for her own good." In the hours and days following each vaccination, my wife and I watched for any one of the many adverse reactions described to us, from the relatively mundane "pain at the injection site" or low-grade fever to the more worrisome febrile seizure (which are convulsions or the loss of consciousness brought on by a fever) to the terrifying threat of ailments like thrombocytopenia (very low levels of platelets in the blood) or acute encephalopathy (brain malfunctions that range in severity from personality changes to coma). After nearly every shot, Annabelle seemed cranky and tired or "fretful," as the CDC describes the temporary condition of approximately half of the children who receive a vaccination. We anxiously anticipated the symptoms detailed in the brightly colored sheets that the nurses handed us as we left our appointments and, after a couple of days, thankfully, Annabelle returned to her normal self.[7]

Fiona's Story

A couple of months after Annabelle was born, I found myself back at the hospital, this time to visit Fiona, the two-year-old daughter of a close friend. Fiona had developed flu-like symptoms, and she quickly grew dehydrated and exhausted. Her parents, Chris and Nickie, had taken her to the emergency room after her fever had spiked and she had grown dangerously dehydrated from diarrhea and vomiting. Fiona was admitted to the hospital after being diagnosed with rotavirus, a nasty illness common among young children whose bodies have not yet developed resistance to it. Rotavirus attacks the lining of the small intestine and causes severe fluid loss, and Fiona was one of the fifty-five thousand children hospitalized in the United States in 2006 after contracting it. It is the most common cause of diarrhea in American children and the leading cause of death among children in developing countries. Worldwide, a child dies every minute from the symptoms of rotavirus. Happily, after several days of isolation, saline I.V.s, and sleep, Fiona fought off the virus and regained her health.[8]

Chris and Nickie never had the option to vaccinate Fiona against rotavirus, because she was a young child during a window of time when there was no available vaccine against it. In 1998, the pharmaceutical company Wyeth had licensed RotaShield, a vaccine against rotavirus, for use in the United States. Clinical trials in the United States, Finland, and Venezuela had shown that the live-attenuated, oral vaccine was highly effective in preventing the severe diarrhea and hospitalization associated with rotavirus. In October 1997, the *New England Journal of Medicine* declared, "The vaccine is safe," although 15 percent of the vaccinated infants had fevers of at least 100.5 degrees within a week after vaccination. Nonetheless, it afforded children 88 percent protection against severe dehydration and a 70 percent reduction in the number of hospital admissions for the symptoms caused by rotavirus.[9]

RotaShield was introduced in the United States in the fall of 1998, and within nine months, fifteen cases of intussusception, a particular type of blockage of the small intestine, appeared among recently vaccinated infants. Intussusception, when it is treated, is rarely fatal, and most of the time it is easily remedied by an enema. About 20 percent of the cases require minor surgery, and the prognosis for children with intussusception who receive medical treatment is very good. The number of cases of intussusception associated with the RotaShield vaccine was minute. In the clinical trials it had shown up less than once in every two thousand cases, but that was still more than twice as frequently as it was found in the control group. The CDC quickly recommended the temporary suspension of the use of RotaShield. Over the next three months, the Vaccine Adverse Events Reporting Systems (VAERS), a vaccine safety surveillance program operated by the U.S. Food and Drug Administration (FDA) and the CDC, reported on data from the one and a half million American children who had received the vaccine. That report, combined with findings in the vaccine's prelicensure clinical evaluation showing an elevated number of cases of intussusception shortly after vaccination, led officials to suspect there was a causal relationship between RotaShield and at least some of these cases of intussusception. In October 1999, by which time fifty-seven cases of intussusception had been identified in recently vaccinated children, the CDC and the U.S. Advisory Committee on Immunization Practices officially withdrew their recommendation for RotaShield, and Wyeth voluntarily withdrew the vaccine from the U.S. market. For the next seven years American infants were unprotected from the threat posed by rotavirus, and in the summer of 2006 Fiona contracted an especially nasty case of it that left her hospitalized for the better part of a week. Annabelle will probably never become as sick from rotavirus as Fiona because she received Merck's RotaTeq vaccine, which was released later in 2006, after clinical trials involving over seventy-two thousand infants in eleven countries did not show an increased risk of intussusception.[10]

Fiona's terrible experience with rotavirus demonstrated to us the potential threat of communicable diseases, and we were thankful that Annabelle had received the RotaTeq vaccine. Nonetheless, there is a striking contrast between our experience with Annabelle's vaccination against hepatitis B and Fiona's inability to be vaccinated against rotavirus. In one case, the public health goal of universal vaccination against hepatitis B led to what we came to believe was the premature administration of a vaccine to a newborn who had no reasonable risk of contracting that particular disease. In the other case, the medical community's prudence and concern to do no harm, along with parents' high expectations for the safety of vaccines, led to removal from the market of a vaccine had been incredibly effective in preventing a common and often lethal illness and that offered a very low risk of a generally nonfatal side effect.

Now It's My Choice

Annabelle is now six, and she has received all of her recommended vaccines—a total of thirty-five different inoculations so far. For her first two dozen (that is, for the first nineteen months of Annabelle's life), my wife and I jointly made the decision of whether to vaccinate her. We were both well-educated, politically moderate professionals, and we trusted our health care providers. We surveyed the claims about vaccines' benefits and risks and talked with our pediatrician about each of the vaccines that Annabelle was scheduled to receive. In browsing the Internet and bookstore offerings, we recognized a fringe movement on the political right that fretted about governmental interference in citizens' personal lives along with another that seemed to emerge from the political left that advocated natural products and worried about the unintended effects of vaccines on children's bodies. The left/right divisions were not at all clear in this controversy, and we often found examples of partisans borrowing and advancing arguments that were more typically offered by authors on the opposite side of the political spectrum.

In addition to the public and political commentaries on vaccines, we read the orthodox medical recommendations from the CDC and from our state's health department. We also read horror stories from vaccine proponents and opponents alike, stories about delicate babies ravaged by communicable diseases as well as accusations from parents who believed their children had been harmed by a vaccine. Finally, we found a substantial body of literature that asserted that the civic responsibility all parents was to vaccinate their children lest they infect the small number of children who could not be vaccinated because they were immunocompromised. Clearly, this was not a topic about which one could be both informed and dispassionate.

We chose to vaccinate Annabelle with all of the recommended vaccines—so far she has been vaccinated against hepatitis B, diphtheria, pertussis, tetanus, polio, pneumococcus, *Haemophilus influenzae* type b, measles, mumps, rubella, varicella, influenza, and rotavirus. But we chose to give them to her one at a time. She was so small and each inoculation was followed by a low-grade fever and general fussiness, so it seemed entirely sensible to space the shots apart by at least a couple of weeks so that we could watch for any severe side effects that she might have to a particular vaccine. That, of course, meant extra trips to the doctor and sometimes a little out-of-pocket expense for insurance copayments, but it seemed like a reasonable thing to do. We found no scientific evidence to validate our concerns about giving her multiple shots at a single visit but plenty of common sense arguments about the capacity of vaccines to overwhelm a baby's body.

When Annabelle was nineteen months old, her mother died. Like the millions of other single parents in the United States, I found myself solely responsible for every decision regarding my daughter's upbringing—decisions like where to send her to school, what opportunities and experiences to provide her, what time she goes to bed, when she can get her ears pierced, and which vaccines (if any) to give her. Somehow, the decision to vaccinate her seemed a lot easier when I had a like-minded partner reinforcing my choice. In addition, I had already begun writing a book on the modern American anti-vaccination movement, and I found myself with a tremendous amount of information and with an intense sense of responsibility. I am no different from any thoughtful and well-informed parent—solo parenting just concentrates these decisions onto one person's shoulders—and I have continued to feel much the same way about vaccines as I did when I had a partner parenting alongside me. I think vaccines are a vital tool in maintaining health and in preventing or substantially limiting outbreaks of troublesome communicable diseases. But I have also continued to be concerned about the growing number of vaccines we give to infants, their unintended consequences, and problems that may arise from our increasing use of them.

Becoming Annabelle's sole surviving parent did not change her vaccination schedule, but it did profoundly change this book. When I began my research in 2007, I had intended to explore the relationship between political ideologies and anxieties about vaccines. I was intrigued by how members of both the political left and the political right in the United States had developed such strikingly strong and similar anxieties about vaccines, and I had hoped to explore the underlying influences in their concerns about vaccines. Over the course of my research—and motivated in no small part by the changes in my family—I came to appreciate that a parent's love owes no allegiance to their politics, even though decisions about a child's healthcare or education might be expressed in terms similar to those used in their discussions about politics. That is, while the political orientation of worried parents most certainly frames their critique of vaccines, anti-vaccination sentiment seems to emerge from something deeper than parents' political perspectives. I have found left- and right-leaning parents borrowing from one another in expressing their concerns about state-mandated vaccines, and I have found staunchly partisan Democrats and Republicans embracing one another's arguments about vaccines across the aisle. Partisans from both sides, in their own way and employing their own terms, exhibit concerns similar to my own about the growing number and potential side effects of our reliance on vaccines. What exactly is it about vaccines that inspires trepidation among Americans?

So, this is a book about something deeper than politics or scientific research. It is a book about something more than just my own experiences, something more inspiring than scientific certainty, and more motivating than a citizen's responsibility to the larger community. This book explores the peculiar context within which modern American parents must make decisions about their children's bodies and reveals a troubling set of problems at the root of parents' current anxieties about vaccines. As both the number of vaccines and the number of vaccine critics has increased, our complicated, confusing, and increasingly contentious environment has grown even more chaotic and bewildering. Never before have we had such capacity to so fundamentally alter our children's bodies and—according to many of the critics of vaccines—their minds. In this book, I hope to put my finger on the source of parents' concerns about vaccines, to understand what exactly makes so many of us anxious about what on the surface seems like such a powerfully good weapon in the public health arsenal. It is my hope that by exploring some of the information available to parents and by examining both the scientific claims and the political issues involved in the modern vaccine debate, I can help other parents who, like me, struggle to do what is best for their children. Unlike many of the decisions we confront in our lives, the decision of whether or not to vaccinate our children is one that we must make, be it by default, rejection, or deliberation. It is a situation like the one that Neal Peart, channeling Ayn Rand, described in Rush's song, *Freewill*: "If you choose not to decide, you still have made a choice." In this case, it is the choice to accept the recommended schedule, to reject it, or to somehow alter it.[11]

This book also has something useful to say to the public health officials who ardently defend the recommended vaccine schedule. I share with them an earnest respect for the capacities of vaccines to protect citizens from deadly and debilitating communicable diseases. I, too, fear the return of childhood scourges like polio and diphtheria, and I recognize how deeply dependent we are on vaccines to prevent epidemics of truly horrible communicable diseases. For parents—who are vested with responsibility first to their child and who are granted the political right to fulfill that responsibility as they see fit—the "big picture" of public health is generally of only secondary concern. Claims about the safety and efficacy (as well as the danger and ineffectiveness) of vaccines are so widespread and wide-ranging that parents are often overwhelmed with information. As an historian of science, someone whose career has been devoted to studying complicated and controversial issues regarding science, medicine, and American society, I can provide some perspective for public health officials as they struggle to find ways to maintain high levels of vaccine compliance in light of the increasing ease with which parents can exempt their children from mandated vaccinations. Because we live in a representative democracy that shows intense respect for individual liberties, and because we have collectively decided that medical decisions ought to be freely made by individuals, not imposed on them, health officials have had to continually adapt their tactics to deal with the public's anxieties about vaccines. Instead of merely offering tactical suggestions to lull parents into compliance and maintain relatively high levels of vaccine coverage, I will uncover for them the source of modern American parents' anxieties about vaccines. Just as parents' reliance on common-sense notions can sometimes lead them astray in making medical decisions, public health officials' notions about the best way to ensure high levels of compliance may very well backfire if they do not realize the true source of parents' concerns.

The book begins with a description of the problem and an overview of the concerns that seem to motivate parents to question the recommended vaccine schedule. We have a very strange situation here: Vaccines are commonly listed among the most valuable tools in the maintenance of the public's health. Their usefulness in decreasing childhood death and lengthening our average lifespan rival or exceed other important public health measures like improved nutrition, antibiotics, and sanitation efforts. Nonetheless, there have always been concerns about injecting healthy people with foreign substances, and lately those concerns have grown more widespread among a group of middle-class, educated Americans. To make matters worse, many state legislatures have responded by loosening the requirements that have brought us closer to universal vaccination. So, we find ourselves in a situation with the most and best vaccines ever available while at the same time a virulent anti-vaccination movement is developing among citizens whom we would otherwise assume to be the most ardent proponents of vaccines. What are we to do?

The second chapter explores the sources of anti-vaccination sentiment that existed in the early 1990s, prior to the full flowering of the movement at the turn of the twenty-first century. It examines the limited opposition to vaccines found among some ideologically motivated Americans of the political left and right prior to the late 1990s. I look at the claims that emerged from many members of the alternative medicine community, who have long expressed concern about vaccines' efficacy and their long-term effects on our health. The concerns introduced by the alternative medicine community in the late twentieth century found their way into mainstream discussion by way of two medical mysteries: the origin of HIV/AIDS and Gulf War Syndrome. The book's second chapter shows how anxieties about vaccines played a role in both of these public health issues. In turn, the mysterious origins of HIV/AIDS and Gulf War Syndrome added fuel to the embers of concern that many Americans already had about vaccines.

In the middle of the book, I describe the origin of the widespread notion that there is a causal link between vaccines and what appears to be an epidemic of autism in the United States. Autism, I argue, has become the battleground on which the struggle between parents' anxieties about vaccines and public health officials' goals of universal vaccination is fought. For parents, the threat of vaccine-induced autism is, in my view, a proxy for a complex set of concerns they have about the modern vaccine schedule, and many parents have seized on it because it provides a ready-made venue for discussing their concerns about vaccines within a group of like-minded advocates. The claim that vaccines might cause or trigger autism emerged in the 1990s from two separate sources—one American and one British—and merged in the public's mind sometime around the turn of the twenty-first century. In the 1970s, 1980s, and 1990s, American public health officials had conducted an aggressive campaign against environmental toxins like lead, mercury, and arsenic. They had a great deal of success in compelling legislation that would limit children's exposure to these dangerous substances and in encouraging parents to rid their homes of them. At the same time, changes in the diagnoses of autism and a substantial increase in public awareness of the disorder generated widespread concern about an apparent autism epidemic in the United States. In the midst of all this, it became known that most childhood vaccines used the preservative thimerosal, which contained mercury. Here was a perfect storm. A large number of parents and some medical professionals connected the apparent autism epidemic, environmental toxins, and vaccines with one another and began assertively questioning the increasingly large number of vaccines routinely given to children, their contents, and their efficacy.

Chapter 4 explores the controversy over autism and the combined vaccine for measles, mumps, and rubella by analyzing the work of Andrew Wakefield, a British surgeon and researcher. In 1998, Wakefield and a dozen of his colleagues at the prestigious Royal Free Hospital in London published an article in the premier British medical journal, the *Lancet*, which suggested a link between the measles, mumps, and rubella (MMR) vaccine and the neurological problems associated with autism. Wakefield had long been interested in intestinal problems like colitis (inflammation of the gastrointestinal tract), and by the mid-1990s he began asserting what he called the "gut-brain link," which hypothesized that certain neurological and developmental disorders might be caused by gastrointestinal ailments that were themselves initiated by some children's bodies' responses to the combined MMR vaccine. When his group published their paper in 1998, Wakefield took their claims a step further by asserting that, until scientists could demonstrate the safety of the combined MMR vaccine, health care providers should give each of the three vaccines separately instead of in the combined form. Wakefield quickly became a pariah in the British medical community and the target of allegations of conflict of interest and ethical misconduct. His claims, however, added to American concerns about environmental toxins and the potential threat posed by some of the components in vaccines. When he immigrated to the United States in 2004, he found a large and supportive constituency among parents of autistic children and among alternative health care providers. Mainstream American health officials have been every bit as critical of him as were their British counterparts, and Wakefield has taken a place at the center of the American controversy over the alleged link between vaccines and autism.

Chapter 5 examines the most vocal American opponents and proponents of vaccines. Under the harsh light of the media and coming from the most polemic figures in the debate, discussions about vaccines—both their potential promise and their peril—are expressed in the most frightening of terms. Jenny McCarthy, a former *Playboy* model and comedian turned actress, author, and activist, is perhaps the best known among the detractors. But vaccines have celebrity supporters as well, including the actress Amanda Peet, along with many ardent supporters from the medical and scientific communities, such as vaccine researcher and advocate Paul Offit. Their rhetoric has fanned the flames of the debate, escalating concerns of both vaccine proponents and detractors.

The book's last chapter offers a description of what in my estimation are the real issues underlying American parents' anxieties about vaccines. Public health officials lament what they take to be "anti-science" attitudes among some members of the public, and they wring their hands over parents' unwillingness to accept what, by now, has become a solid medical consensus against claims of a link between autism and vaccines. In a vain attempt to quiet the storm, they attack any public figure willing to openly state some of the concerns that millions of Americans hold. In doing so, they are simply treating the symptoms of the problem. Anxieties about vaccines are, I believe, indicators of a set of underlying problems, and in the book's final chapter I lay out what I see as the issues that really need to be addressed—or at least admitted—if we are to continue to see the high rates of vaccine compliance we enjoy today.

Finally, I conclude with what I believe is a potential way forward for parents and policy-makers alike. It is not a manifesto of any sort or even a checklist of priorities. Rather, it is the promotion of a worldview that recognizes the potential value of vaccines, the economic and public health pressures that continue to lengthen the list of mandated and recommended vaccines, and the responsibilities we have to our children and to one another. We must also acknowledge that ultimately parents—not scientists, physicians, or politicians—have the choice to vaccinate their children or to refuse vaccinations. Parents' vaccine anxieties are a symptom of deeper problems, and no amount of debate, scientific evidence, or celebrity endorsement will make these problems go away. We can begin to address parents' anxieties and perhaps resolve this dilemma only after we recognize the bases for parents' concerns. For better or for worse, scientists or physicians alone cannot assuage our worries about vaccines with their research results or their professional authority. Vaccine-anxious parents are motivated by deeply felt concerns about the modern American vaccine schedule that must be understood and addressed. This book attempts to uncover the source of those concerns, explain the evolution of the controversy, and move us past the proxy debate over vaccines and autism that has dominated the discussion since the turn of the century.

1

Risk and Reward

Annabelle, Fiona, and the millions of other American children born over the last twenty years have received an unprecedented number of vaccines. Between 1983 and 2005, the number of diseases against which children are routinely vaccinated doubled, and the number of mandated and recommended vaccinations tripled. New vaccines are added to states' lists of mandated vaccines through a process that begins with the Centers for Disease Control and Prevention's Advisory Committee on Immunization Practices. The committee, made up of fifteen members drawn from the scientific and medical communities, meets three times a year. It offers official recommendations for the use of vaccines to be adopted by state legislatures and by physicians. But it is up to individual state legislatures to adopt the committee's recommendations and make a particular vaccine mandatory, and it is up to pediatricians to recommend vaccines that are not on their states' lists of mandated vaccines to their patients' parents.[1]

A century ago, children received only the smallpox vaccine. By the early 1980s, vaccines for diphtheria, pertussis, tetanus (administered together in the DPT vaccine), polio, and measles, mumps, and rubella (administered together in the MMR vaccine) were developed and adopted in most states as mandatory (table 1). Over the last twenty years, six more vaccines were added to the list along with the annual influenza vaccine. Today, by the time they are six years old, fully vaccinated American children receive about three dozen immunizations consisting of nearly fifty vaccines (table 2). At the same time, vaccine compliance rates are at record highs. In 2007, among two- and three-year-olds in the United States, vaccine coverage topped 90 percent each for polio, measles, mumps, rubella, *Haemophilus influenzae* type b, hepatitis B, varicella, and pneumococcus. Today, over 80 percent of American three-year-olds have received all of their state-mandated vaccines. At the opening of the twenty-first century, more children are receiving far more vaccines than ever before in American history.[2]

Table 1.   Diseases the CDC Recommends Children Be Vaccinated against
by Age Six, 1983 and 2008

	1983	2008
	Diphtheria	Diphtheria
	Pertussis	Pertussis
	Tetanus	Tetanus
	Polio	Polio
	Measles	Measles
	Mumps	Mumps
	Rubella	Rubella
		Hepatitis A
		Hepatitis B
		Rotavirus
		Haemophilus influenzae type B
		Pneumococcus
		Annual influenza
		Varicella
Total number of diseases	7	14

Along with the rapidly growing number of vaccines have come increasing worries among parents about the number of shots, their frequency, and the possible unintended negative consequences. Lately we have seen escalating concerns among Americans about pharmaceutical companies putting profitability before safety as well as fears about the potentially harmful effects of the medical community's one-size-fits-all approach to vaccinations. Criticism of vaccines is coming from both ends of the political spectrum and from points in between. Left-leaning parents mingle concerns about vaccines with their environmental activism, health-conscious lifestyles, and anxieties about corporate power and profit motives. They are joined by rightwing libertarians who dislike governmental interference with what they consider personal decisions and by conspiracy theorists that see in vaccines a government plot to oppress or eliminate certain segments of the population. Individuals who might be political rivals on other issues frequently borrow from one another in making their arguments. Add to that the incredible amount of information on the subject now available through a variety of media outlets including the Internet—much of it unfiltered by accredited experts and repeated by various celebrity advocates—and you have an entire generation of parents

Table 2. Vaccines Recommended by the CDC from Birth to Age Six, 1983 and 2008

	1983	2008
	DPT (2 mo.)	Hepatitis B (birth)
	Polio (2 mo.)	Hepatitis B (1–2 mo.)
	DPT (4 mo.)	Rotavirus (2 mo.)
	Polio (3 mo.)	DTaP (2 mo.)
	DPT (6 mo.)	*Haemophilus influenzae* type B (2 mo.)*
	MMR (15 mo.)	Pneumococcus (2 mo.)
	DPT (18 mo.)	Polio (2 mo.)*
	Polio (18 mo.)	*Haemophilus influenzae* type B (4 mo.)†
	DPT (4–6 yr)	Pneumococcus (4 mo.)
		DTaP (4 mo.)
		Polio (4 mo.)*
		Rotavirus (4 mo.)
		Influenza (6 mo.)
		DTaP (6 mo.)
		Haemophilus influenzae type B (6 mo.)*
		Pneumococcus (6 mo.)
		Hepatitis B (6–18 mo.)
		Polio (6–18 mo.)*
		Rotavirus (8 mo.)
		Varicella (12–15 mo.)†
		Hepatitis A (12–15 mo.)
		Haemophilus influenzae type B (12–15 mo.)*
		Pneumococcus (12–15 mo.)
		MMR (12–15 mo.)
		DTaP (15–18 mo.)
		Influenza (18 mo.)
		Hepatitis A (18–24 mo.)
		Influenza (2–3 yr)
		Influenza (3–4 yr)
		Influenza (4–5 yr)
		Polio (4–6 yr)*
		DTaP (4–6 yr)
		MMR (4–6 yr)
		Varicella (4–6 yr)†
		Influenza (5–6 yr)
Total number of inoculations	10	26 to 35

*This can be combined with the DTaP vaccine in the DTaP-IPV/Hib vaccine to reduce the overall number of vaccinations in the first six years of life by seven.

†This can be combined with the MMR vaccine in the MMRV vaccine to reduce the overall number of vaccinations in the first six years of life by two.

who are apprehensive about what public health authorities herald as the single most effective tool in preventing communicable diseases.

Parents are not merely talking about their concerns about vaccines, they are acting on them. A large and growing number of parents are choosing not to vaccinate their children with one or more of the mandated vaccines. Today, 40 percent of American parents have chosen to delay or refuse a recommended or mandated vaccine for their children. To make matters worse, public health officials have found pockets of very low vaccine compliance in various places around the country, some with high numbers of unvaccinated children. For example, in the public schools on Vashon Island, located a short ferry ride from Seattle, Washington, 18 percent of students are exempted from a mandated vaccine. Similar hotbeds of vaccine exemptions include Boulder, Colorado, and Ashland, Oregon, where on average 28.1 percent of students are exempt from one or more vaccines. In some Ashland schools, exemptions for particular vaccines are as high as 66.7 percent. These parents are not simply forgetting to have their children vaccinated, nor are they too poor to have access to health care; they are making conscious decisions not to vaccinate their children with one or more of the mandated vaccines.

The clustering of these exemptions raises concern among public health officials about their potential to generate disease outbreaks that can spread to children in other areas. In addition to the children whose parents have chosen not to vaccinate them, there are many children who are not vaccinated because they have medical exemptions and many others who, despite being vaccinated, have lost their immunity over time and are susceptible to communicable disease. In 2008, public health officials singled out Washington State for its high number of unvaccinated children and identified the source of one of the largest outbreaks in recent history of measles as an unvaccinated child who spread the disease to seven other unvaccinated children in her household. Health authorities see intentionally unvaccinated children as threats to everyone, recognizing that vaccines' efficacy wanes over time and that in some cases even vaccinated children are still capable of contracting diseases. Some officials warn that "difficult decisions may need to be made to deny exceptions . . . in order to avoid a snowballing of exceptions that would threaten not only those who seek exemption, but some percentage of those who undergo vaccination."[3]

The public discussion about vaccines has grown so complicated and confusing that one can easily find competing claims about nearly every vaccine-related fact or event. For example, both the proponents and the detractors of the mandatory vaccination schedule have used the case of the introduction and withdrawal of RotaShield to support their positions. Vaccine advocates have pointed to the high levels of safety expected of vaccines—after all, an investigation into the vaccine began after only fifteen reports of intussusception among recently vaccinated children. Detractors see this case as an example of corruption and lax standards. In 2000, a majority staff report from the U.S. House Committee on Government Reform reported that the vaccine was approved and sent to market even though an increased number of intussusception cases appeared during the prelicensure trials of RotaShield. This was perhaps because, as the report asserted, the "conflict of interest rules employed by the FDA and the CDC have been weak, enforcement has been lax, and committee members with substantial ties to pharmaceutical companies have been given waivers to participate in committee proceedings." Critics of vaccination programs draw from the report to assert that, despite the prelicensure cases of intussusception among children vaccinated with RotaShield, the vaccine was approved because "four out of eight CDC advisory committee members who voted to approve guidelines for the vaccine in June 1998 had financial ties to pharmaceutical companies that were developing different versions of the vaccine. Additionally, three out of five FDA advisory committee members who voted to approve the rotavirus vaccine in December 1997 had financial ties to pharmaceutical companies that were developing different versions of the vaccine."

In response, public health officials have become increasingly concerned with managing the media's response to research results, and they have made changes to vaccine policy in hopes of avoiding a loss in the public's confidence in a particular vaccine or in vaccines generally. Some recognize that maintaining high levels of vaccine compliance requires better educating the public about the side effects from vaccines as well as enhancing appreciation for the long-term benefits of mandated vaccines.[4] Nonetheless, little effort has been put forward by health officials to address Americans' concerns about what on the surface seems like serious conflict of interest problems in the research, manufacture, and administration of vaccines in the United States.

To bolster public confidence in the value of vaccines, proponents remind the public about the serious threat of communicable diseases and the success the medical community has had in nearly eliminating many of the most deadly diseases. As part of their efforts to educate the public about efficacy of vaccines, the Vaccine Education Center at the Children's Hospital of Philadelphia tells parents, "Vaccines have literally transformed the landscape of medicine over the course of the twentieth century." According to their website, before vaccines were developed for certain communicable diseases, parents in the United States could expect that every year:

- Polio would paralyze ten thousand children.
- Rubella (German measles) would cause birth defects and mental retardation in as many as twenty thousand newborns.
- Measles would infect about four million children, killing three thousand.
- Diphtheria would be one of the most common causes of death in school-aged children.
- A bacterium called *Haemophilus influenzae* type b (Hib) would cause meningitis in fifteen thousand children, leaving many with permanent brain damage.
- Pertussis (whooping cough) would kill thousands of infants.

In 1996, the CDC studied the efficacy of vaccines in reducing the incidence of vaccine-preventable diseases. It found that since the introduction of vaccines for rubella, diphtheria, *Haemophilus influenzae* type b, measles, mumps, pertussis, polio, and tetanus, we have seen a drop of between 97.8 percent and 100 percent in each of the diseases.[5]

Even the most ardent proponents of vaccines also recognize that the administration of any vaccine carries with it some risk of undesirable side effects that range from mild discomfort to—in very rare cases—disability or death. The CDC, for example, states, "Immunizations, like any medication, can cause adverse events." Likewise, the Vaccine Education Center explains that every vaccine has negative consequences for some of the children who receive them: "Almost all vaccines can cause pain, redness or tenderness at the site of injection. And some vaccines cause more severe side effects." These include high fevers, seizures, comas, swelling of the brain, severe infection at the injection site, life-threatening allergic reactions, pneumonia, permanent brain damage, major organ system failure, intussusception, deafness, and even diseases like Guillain-Barré Syndrome. However, as public health officials are quick to point out, such reactions are exceptionally rare, occurring far less often than the diseases against which the vaccines protect had occurred. This allows a vaccine to be declared safe because each vaccine's "benefits must clearly and definitively outweigh its risks." Moreover, despite their shared use of the term "risk," parents and health officials may have fundamentally different notions of how to weigh it in making health care decisions. While health officials work with a sample size of thousands or even millions, parents consider risks one child at a time. In discussions about vaccine safety, it is common to hear parents say, "What if your child is that one in a million?"[6]

Of more concern to most parents than the risk-benefit analysis inherent to each vaccine is the larger and increasingly complicated question of how many vaccines we ought to administer to ourselves and to our children. Recent polls of parents have found that, while most appreciate the capacity of vaccines to help maintain children's health, they were nonetheless concerned about the rapidly increasing numbers of vaccines that their children were expected to receive. A poll of parents in the year 2000 found that 87 percent "deemed immunization an extremely important action that parents can take to keep their children well," but a third "believed that children get more immunizations than are good for them." Only four years later, another poll found that almost 90 percent of surveyed parents expressed concerns about the number of diseases against which children were vaccinated, while only 14 percent questioned any individual vaccine's efficacy. The elimination of polio or hepatitis B is doubtlessly desirable, and the vaccines against such deadly and debilitating communicable diseases have been incredibly effective. More recently adopted vaccines, however, target far less common or much less serious ailments like the once common and rarely deadly chickenpox infection. Nonetheless, the vaccine against chickenpox is mandated alongside vaccines for deadly diseases like measles and diphtheria.[7]

Further complicating the situation are the justifications and sales pitches for some new vaccines. For example, parents are frequently told that the varicella vaccine, which protects against the chickenpox, should be administered because it prevents inconvenience to the parent and child. "Even with uncomplicated cases," the CDC's website states, "children with chickenpox miss an average of five to six days of school, and parents or other caregivers miss three to four days of work to care for sick children." The American Academy of Pediatrics employs the same argument, but with different numbers, asserting that "parents may have to miss work while their children are home from school or child care. In the average household, a child with chickenpox misses eight or nine days of school, and adult caretakers lose up to two days of work." Similarly, the American Academy of Family Physicians asserts, "Because of the lost time from work, chickenpox can be a significant cost to parents of children who get the illness."[8]

The message to parents is clear: The inconvenience and financial costs of missing work can easily be avoided by simply agreeing to have your pediatrician administer the varicella vaccine to your child. Such an approach smacks of an easy techno-fix for a complex social and economic dilemma. In this case, the vaccine reduces the problem created by an economic and cultural system that penalizes a parent for having to stay home from work to take care of a sick child. Some vaccines initiate criticism of so-called pharmacological techno-fixes for what detractors consider to be personal or social shortcomings. The ardent search for a vaccine to protect against HIV/AIDS, the promotion of the vaccine for the human papillomavirus (HPV), and the mandated vaccination for hepatitis B are all targets for critics who claim that the vaccines protect against diseases that are caused primarily by unprotected sexual activity. Instead of engaging in the arduous task of altering people's behaviors, these vaccines, with the ease of a few simple shots, would do away with what moralists consider the natural consequences of problematic behaviors.[9]

The vaccine for varicella (popularly known as the chickenpox) has been the subject of a great deal of controversy recently as research has indicated that the vaccine does not provide the same kind of lifelong immunity provided by contracting the disease. This suggests that children may be protected against the disease while they are young but are left vulnerable as they become adults. As age increases, chickenpox becomes an increasingly serious ailment; by the 1980s, adults accounted for only 2 percent of the cases of chickenpox but were among nearly 50 percent of the small handful of people who died from complications associated with the disease. In 2007, research published in the *New England Journal of Medicine* concluded that the protection offered by the varicella vaccine waned after about five years, and a second dose of the vaccine "could improve protection from both primary vaccine failure and waning vaccine-induced immunity." According to a Reuters interview with the authors of the study, "No one knows how long the effects of the second shot would last." To make matters worse, shortly before the study was published, Merck had released its new MMRV vaccine, ProQuad, which added the vaccine against the chickenpox to the existing MMR vaccine. The new combined MMRV vaccine effectively reduced parents' ability to choose to vaccinate against diseases like the measles without also having to vaccinate against the chickenpox; this gave parents another reason to be apprehensive about the current vaccine regime.[10]

Efforts to increase the uptake of particular vaccines have, at times, jeopardized public support of vaccines. Take, for example, Merck's Gardasil, which protects against four strains of the human papillomavirus, two of which are associated with cervical cancer and two of which cause genital warts. Gardasil was the subject of contentious debate in 2006 and 2007 when Merck's lobbyists pressed state legislatures to include it on their lists of mandated vaccines. The issue came to a head in February 2007, when the Republican governor of Texas, Rick Perry, sidestepped the usual legislative process for adding vaccines to his state's list of mandated vaccines; he issued an executive order requiring all Texas girls to be vaccinated with Gardasil. Three weeks later the Associated Press reported that Perry's aides had crafted the executive order on the same day that Merck had donated $5,000 to Perry's campaign. It was also learned that Perry's former chief of staff was by then a lobbyist for Merck and that the governor had accepted $6,000 from the company during his previous reelection campaign. In May, amid considerable public pressure, the state legislature passed a bill that overturned Perry's executive order.[11]

Controversies like the one in Texas led to a passionate response from advocacy groups and public health experts, and Merck eventually abandoned its lobbying efforts to get Gardasil included on the list of state-mandated vaccines. The *New York Times* reported "the company said it made the decision after realizing that its lobbying campaign had fueled objections across the country that could undermine adoption of the vaccine." As Merck withdrew its lobbyists, it set its advertising agency to work creating direct-to-consumer advertisements that ran on television, in movie theaters, and in many mass-market magazines. Campaigns for the drug featured a sophisticated website. Merck's extensive "I Choose" and "One Less" campaigns urge women to protect themselves and their underage daughters against cervical cancer and some strains of HPV without ever discussing sexual issues or explaining that HPV is a common virus that is almost always harmless. No longer merely instruments of public health, such recently released vaccines have taken their place alongside other enhancement pharmaceuticals that promise to improve the quality of individuals' lives by allowing them freedom from inconveniences like missed work days or safe sex practices.[12]

Vaccine proponents have worried about the politicization of vaccines as increasing numbers of parents lobby state legislatures to loosen the process to obtain exemptions. Merck has taken advantage of the political controversy over its aggressive lobbying efforts to attract more consumers. Instead of relying on state legislatures to add their HPV vaccine to the list of mandated vaccines, they have marketed Gardasil to a particular ideological category of Americans. Just as Toyota solicits environmentally conscientious consumers with the Prius, Merck has worked to attract politically progressive parents to Gardasil with advertisements that urge them to take advantage of the opportunity to protect their children, boys and girls alike, from the four strains of HPV that are most commonly associated with cervical cancer and genital warts. In this context, Merck has profited from the notion that the only significant opposition to mandating Gardasil came from members of the religious right. Merck has capitalized on the political controversy over Gardasil—perhaps even to the point of perpetuating or enhancing it—which is problematic in light of recent studies concluding that pharmaceutical companies like Merck spend almost twice as much money on advertising as they do on research and development. Moreover, these pharmaceutical companies use direct-to-consumer advertising methods for drugs that are only available by prescription.[13]

The vaccines against varicella and HPV are the two newest to be added to the list of mandated (in the case of varicella) and recommended (in the case of HPV) vaccines, and they are the two that seem to most frequently elicit parents' concerns. In a recent survey, among those parents who have refused to allow their pediatricians to administer a vaccine, the HPV and varicella vaccines were the two most commonly refused. When asked about their concerns, more than three-quarters of the parents who refused the HPV vaccine said they did so because not enough research had been done on it, and because it had not been on the market long enough. In the case of the varicella vaccine, most parents (78 percent) said they would prefer that their child get chickenpox than be vaccinated against it.[14]

What Worries Us?

Public health officials and medical authorities see tremendous promise in vaccines and give unwavering support for universal vaccination efforts. Any criticism of vaccines is especially worrisome for them. In response to challenges to the safety or efficacy of vaccines they often—and regrettably—raise the issue of religion as a convenient explanation for parents' concerns. In fact, very few people refrain from vaccinating their children for formal religious justifications. Nationally, only about one percent of children are exempted from vaccinations for religious reasons. Nonetheless, descriptions of anti-vaccinators from public health officials generally make allusions to religious objections to vaccination. To be sure, some parents without religious objections to vaccines avoid vaccinating their children by employing religious exemptions, either out of convenience or because it is the only avenue for a sanctioned exemption in their state. It is also likely that public health officials' notions are overly informed by historical memory. They overemphasize the century-old religious objections to vaccines while overlooking the more recent concerns that have little to do with formal or informal religious resistance to compulsory vaccination. Aside from tiny fringe fundamentalist healing sects, no significant American religious group categorically disallows its followers from being vaccinated. A cultural tendency among members of some groups—like the Amish, Jehovah's Witnesses, and Christian Scientists—encourages skepticism about mandated vaccines. However, these groups make up only a tiny fraction of the American population.[15]

Health care providers and public health officials also frequently assert that the number of vaccine skeptics has increased because as diseases occur less frequently, parents have grown apathetic about the potential threat of these vaccine-controlled diseases. As Mark Sawyer, a pediatrician and infectious disease specialist at Rady Children's Hospital in San Diego explains, "The very success of immunizations has turned out to be an Achilles' heel. Most of these parents have never seen measles, and don't realize it could be a bad disease so they turn their concerns to unfounded risks. They do not perceive risk of the disease but perceive risk of the vaccine." Elsewhere, in an analysis of parents who opposed compulsory vaccination, researchers asserted, "Because many parents lack firsthand knowledge of vaccine-preventable diseases such as measles or polio, they are not likely to perceive such illnesses to be an immediate threat to the health of their children." This assertion was validated, researchers say, by a 1999 telephone survey that found parents were more likely to refuse a vaccine when they perceived the severity of the disease to be low.[16]

From a parent's point of view, none of the explanations commonly offered by the medical community adequately addresses the anxiety I feel vaccinating my daughter. First, I have no religious or moral impulses about vaccines. I recognize that some are made with animal products, and some were developed with the use of aborted fetuses. These facts alone do not prevent me from allowing them to be administered to my daughter. Furthermore, I fully understand that diseases like measles and diphtheria are terribly dangerous, especially to young children. Recent polls demonstrate that the vast majority of American parents likewise recognize that children need vaccines for diseases that are no longer common. Not personally knowing any children who have had these diseases in no way alleviates my appreciation of their threat to Annabelle. There are countless precautions I take against real and perceived threats to her safety—from baby proof latches on cupboard doors and expensive car seats to tossing out her plastic baby bottles when I learned about the potential threat of bisphenol A and spending the extra money to buy organic foods. Just as I know of no children who have been harmed by measles or diphtheria, I know of none who has been seriously harmed by the contents of cupboards or by plastic baby bottles. Nonetheless, I am concerned about the capacity of these things to harm my daughter, and I have taken what I believe are sufficient precautions to preserve her health, as the bottles of hand sanitizer I stash in my glove box and briefcase testify. The threat of communicable diseases, in fact, looms large in my mind, and any claims that I fail to appreciate the peril they represent to Annabelle are simply wrong.[17]

There is, moreover, a significant difference between safeguards like baby proofing my home and vaccinating my child: unlike most of the measures I take to protect Annabelle, vaccines come with a recognized risk of side effects. There are no potential adverse side effects other than to my wallet of organic foods, safety latches, or costly car seats. Because more vaccines means more potential side effects, parents are growing increasingly concerned about the rapidly increasing number of vaccines that they are expected to allow pediatricians to administer to their children. It is not merely the nature of vaccines that disturbs parents; it is their sheer number. American children are now expected to get between twenty-six and thirty-five inoculations by the time they start kindergarten. To make matters worse, three-quarters of these vaccinations are administered in the first eighteen months of life, with as many as six at a single office visit. Every new vaccine added to the vaccine schedule adds yet another batch of potential side effects.

Parents' concerns about vaccines extend beyond a simple recognition of benefits and risks, and public health officials need to appreciate how a parent thinks about the potential benefits and dangers offered by vaccines. Most parents are much more willing to accept the consequences of a communicable disease than they are willing to accept the consequences of having made a child sick by giving them a vaccine. Guilt by omission—failing to administer a vaccine and as a result a child contracts a communicable disease—seems preferable to guilt by commission—making a child sick as a result of an adverse reaction to a vaccine. This attitude was nicely demonstrated in the "Readers' Comments" section of the *New York Times* website in response to a story on personal-belief exemptions for vaccines. Wendell Jones of Albuquerque, New Mexico, wrote, "A part of the emotional equation for parents is the difference between consequences resulting from 'acts of God' (like coming down with measles) and those resulting from actions on my part (like developing a condition from receiving a vaccination). As a parent, I can more easily live with the first than with the second." Similarly, in *The Vaccine Book: Making the Right Choice for Your Child*, Robert Sears described his experience with a parent who said that she would rather risk having her children contracting a disease than risk causing a side effect from vaccinating them because, "If her children suffer a severe course of a disease, it won't be because of something she did. Rather, it will be because of something she didn't do. She said that she would rather live with that type of choice."[18]

Health authorities' efforts to maintain public vigilance against vaccine-preventable diseases have led them to describe the potential threat posed by vaccine-preventable communicable disease in near hysterical terms. Readers frequently see the term *epidemic* used in descriptions of minor outbreaks of diseases, and vaccine proponents describe parents who refuse to vaccinate their children against particular diseases as *free-riders* or *parasites* because they benefit from the inoculated majority. In both Great Britain and the United States, public health officials routinely describe the threat of a measles epidemic given the supposedly falling rates of vaccination that are claimed to be caused by concerns about vaccines. For example, in 2008, the CDC reported a spike in the number of confirmed measles cases. During the first six months of the year, there were several small outbreaks in Illinois, New York, and Washington State that brought the total number of confirmed cases for the first half of the year to 131, more than twice what Americans had seen in the previous year but not substantially outside the range of confirmed cases typical over the previous two decades. Given that the United States was also experiencing record high vaccination rates and that vaccine-preventable childhood disease deaths were at a record low, there was no real cause for concern. Nonetheless, the press reported, "pediatricians and health experts are sounding the alarm, noting that measles, which is virulently contagious, is the first disease to crop up when vaccination rates fall." It may well be true that we would see an increase in measles cases *if* vaccination rates dropped; however, a slight increase in cases over the previous several years was not the result of a drop in vaccination rates.[19]

In 2008, in hopes of reenergizing public concern about communicable diseases and fighting what it called "preparedness fatigue," the CDC introduced the Pandemic Influenza Storybook, an online collection of personal recollections from survivors, families, and friends of victims of the 1918 flu pandemic. "Complacency is enemy number one when it comes to preparing for another influenza pandemic," explained CDC director Julie Gerberding. The stories "serve as a sobering reminder of the devastating impact that influenza can have, and reading them is a must for anyone involved in public health preparedness."[20]

Claims about how the reduced incidence of communicable diseases has altered parents' thinking about the benefits and risks of vaccines are only half right. It is not the case that parents merely do not appreciate the danger of communicable diseases. Instead, the population-wide reduction in the incidence of these diseases has helped to alter parents' calculus in making decisions about vaccinating their children because it has altered the amount of risk parents are willing to take in the name of prevention. The 1999 telephone poll that found a relationship between parents' perception of the likelihood of their children contracting a particular communicable disease, the perceived severity of a disease, and their attitudes about compulsory vaccination provides us with ample evidence of this change. Parents were most likely to refuse vaccines against the diseases that were actually the least immediately threatening to their children (like the chickenpox and hepatitis B), and least likely to refuse vaccines against the most immediately threatening diseases (such as Hib, polio, and measles).

So, let us be clear here: vaccines are not "victims of their own success," because the reduced incidence in communicable disease has not lessened concern about particular communicable diseases any more than the invention of airbags or the availability of safer car seats has reduced my concern that Annabelle will be injured in an automobile accident. If anything, the reduction in the prevalence of communicable diseases has heightened my concern to protect her against them, which follows what appears to be a generally lower tolerance among Americans for risk to their children generally. In the context of reduced tolerance for risk, parents have grown increasingly concerned not only about communicable diseases, but also about the potential short- and long-term side effects of the intensive vaccination regime.[21]

Vaccines and Values

One good explanation of the tensions that have emerged between parents and public health officials can be found in the work of scholars of rhetoric and argumentation. Rhetoricians have described how participants on either side of an argument work from a set of agreed upon values about important claims, ideas, or goals. In scientific arguments, discussion and agreement about these values are generally confined to the early formulations of the concepts and rules that will govern the argument. That is most certainly the case with discussions about vaccines among medical professionals and in their public statements in support of official vaccine recommendations. The mutually agreed upon value of widespread public health—the largest benefit for the largest number of people—motivates their ardent promotion of vaccination for every citizen who is not deemed too immunocompromised to shoulder the relatively low risk of adverse side effects. However, in fields like law, politics, and philosophy, rhetoricians tell us that consideration of values occurs at all stages of the development and execution of an argument. We see this in debates over vaccines, as worried parents and vaccine detractors launch attacks on the medical orthodoxy over everything from the contents of vaccines and their efficacy to the safety studies before new vaccines are put on the market, the timing of their administration, and their long-term effects. While parents and public health officials may hold many values in common, their value hierarchies are sometimes at odds, and the rules by which they wage arguments often differ considerably. The result is a chaotic environment in which, parents, not public health authorities, ultimately decide whether or not to vaccinate children.[22]

It is not simply that parents and health officials do not agree on the relevant values or on an acceptable value hierarchy, they also engage fundamentally different sorts of values when considering the issues surrounding vaccines. Rhetoricians distinguish between two types of values: abstract values, like truth, justice, or beauty that exist only as concepts and concrete values, which are attached to specific tangible things, like a particular virus. Parents necessarily grapple with a diverse collection of abstract values when they consider the benefits and risks—both to their children and to society at large—and decide for or against particular vaccines. Paramount among these abstract values is their children's health, which is an illimitable, perpetually improvable value that cannot be judged against some normative standard of health, but only against parents' perception of how much healthier or less healthy that child might have otherwise been. This is what is happening when someone says, "My mother smoked when she carried me, and I turned out healthy," and another replies, "Yes, but how much healthier might you have been had she not smoked?" There is no normative standard of health when we think about our children or even about our own childhoods. Instead, we can only imagine how much better or worse our current health might be had something been done differently.[23]

While parents struggle to rank competing abstract values, in discussions about vaccines and vaccine compliance, public health officials have found a way to transform the abstract value of public health into a concrete value by quantifying it. By tracking the number of diagnoses of a particular disease and by virtue of their collective acceptance that the absence of any diagnoses of a disease is equivalent to health, they have transformed the abstract value of public health into a concrete value. Their adamant assertion that the benefits of vaccines far outweigh their risks is possible only because medical authorities have generated a normative standard of health, which they measure by recording the number of diagnoses of a particular disease. Unlike the parent who is forever vexed with the question of "how much healthier might my child have been had I done (or not done) X," public health officials can reach the point of perfect health in fighting a particular disease when the number of diagnoses drops to zero, as it did in the 1970s with smallpox, for which a vaccine is no longer necessary. Their concrete value of health emerges as a product of public health statistics, which allow the medical community a level of certainty about the overall goodness of vaccines that is simply not available to parents.[24]

We conclude, therefore, with a curious dilemma: how is it that a fantastically successful instrument of public health, a cheap intervention that has saved millions of lives and prevented unimaginable illness and disability, has become the target of such virulent contention? How is it that something so obviously beneficial to children's well being has become the source of so much anxiety for parents? More specifically, how—as either a parent or a public health official—does one navigate this controversy and make the best decisions for our children?

Abandoning for now my perspective as a parent and taking up the tools of an historian of science and medicine, I hope to show how the modern American controversy over vaccines emerged in the 1990s and how it has evolved over the last two decades. There is a substantial history of opposition to mandatory vaccination, beginning in England with Reverend Edmund Massey's 1772 sermon, "The Dangerous and Sinful Practice of Inoculation." Massey argued that the diseases that might be prevented by vaccines were in fact God's tools for punishing sinners. Public resistance to vaccines grew rapidly after Britain began requiring the vaccination of all infants in 1853 for smallpox, and anti-vaccination sentiment was imported into the United States by the prominent British anti-vaccinationist William Tebb in 1879.[25]

Regardless of the claims made by vaccine proponents, eighteenth- and nineteenth-century vaccine controversies have little direct impact on my and other parents' concerns about current vaccine policy. Modern vaccine anxieties have nothing to do with Massey's notions of a vengeful God, nor are they shaped by particular religious objections to the way in which vaccines are researched or manufactured. It may well be that public health officials can find past challenges to vaccines that seem similar to some of today's claims about vaccines. They might even find some short-term solutions to the problem of parents' declining commitment to universal vaccination. However, modern vaccine anxieties are different from those expressed in the past because both the vaccines and the contexts are vastly different. It might be heretical for an historian to argue this, but the historical memory of centuries-old British and American anti-vaccination campaigns looms too large in the minds of today's public health officials. It distorts their notions about modern parents' apprehension about vaccines and makes them ineffective at addressing concerns that can quickly and easily erode away the high compliance rates for vaccines we now enjoy.

The modern American vaccine controversy finds its origins in the 1990s. It is firmly rooted in the educated American middle class—the *New York Times*–reading parents, as one of my colleagues called them—and most public health officials oversimplify the complexity of today's parents' concerns. To understand the modern American vaccine controversy, we need to identify precisely who worries about vaccines and why so many American parents intentionally avoid vaccinating their children despite the substantial pressure to vaccinate.[26]

Anti-Vaccinators, the Under-Vaccinated, and the Vaccine-Anxious Parent

Who are these vaccine skeptics and how do they express their concerns about vaccines? First, let us recognize that the majority of the children in the United States whom the CDC describes as "under-vaccinated" are not the children of parents who have conscientiously chosen not to vaccinate their children. Data from 2001 show more than a third of all American children under the age of three have not received all of their mandated vaccines. In 2008, estimated rates of complete vaccine compliance among two-year olds vary from as low as 58.5 percent (Idaho) to as high as 79.6 percent (New Hampshire). This means that in any given state between 20 percent and 40 percent of children are under-vaccinated. The majority of the American children who have fewer than the recommended and mandated number of vaccinations are not intentionally unvaccinated; rather, they are children who have slipped through the many gaping cracks in our health care system. They are often poor and uninsured, and their status as under-vaccinated generally mirrors the low level of health care to which they have had access. These children deserve significant attention from all of us, but they are not the subject of this book.[27]

The objects of my attention, instead, are the growing number of children whose parents have intentionally prevented them from being vaccinated or have chosen to delay one or more of the mandated or recommended vaccines until their children were older than the recommended age for a particular vaccine. The most recent polling data show that 11.5 percent of American parents have consciously refused vaccines that their pediatricians have recommended, and about twice as many more parents have intentionally delayed a recommended or mandated vaccination for their children. Official religious and philosophical exemptions account for only 0.1 percent (Arkansas) to 6.8 percent (Minnesota) of the total number of under-vaccinated children in the United States. This means that most of the parents who chose to avoid fully vaccinating their children have taken advantage of the gaps in the administrative oversight in the system. Public health authorities leave it to school and daycare officials to enforce vaccine mandates, and parents can often go months or years without any need to account for their children's missed vaccines. For children who are too young to attend school or those not in a daycare, there are no institutionalized compulsions for them to be vaccinated.[28]

A sizable proportion of the nearly 40 percent of parents who have chosen to alter or reject the recommended schedule includes mothers who are older than thirty years of age. It appears that mothers over the age of forty are especially prone to concern about vaccines, perhaps because they are more savvy consumers of medical care or are more unlikely or unwilling to be deferential to medical authorities. In contrast to public health officials' assumption that ignorance plays a significant role in under-vaccination, women with college educations were more likely to delay or reject some of the recommended vaccines than were their lesser-educated peers. A 2007 survey found that college-educated women were 16 percent more likely to have children who lacked all their recommended vaccinations than were women who had no college education whatsoever. White parents question the vaccine schedule more frequently than do parents of color, and parents who live in the western region of the United States are more likely than their peers elsewhere in the country to reject or delay recommended vaccines. Hispanic parents rarely reject or delay vaccines, although they are among the most concerned of all demographic groups about the potential serious adverse effects of vaccines. Most of the parents who choose not to fully vaccinate their children appear to have poor relationships with their children's health care providers, even when they generally seem to have positive feelings about traditional medical care. When asked about their specific concerns, the parents who expressed doubts about vaccines are most worried about the safety of vaccines and about potential adverse side effects. The varicella vaccine, more than any other vaccine, prompted parents to question the entirety of the vaccine schedule.[29]

The claims expressed by modern American anti-vaccinators, by the parents who choose to forgo or delay certain vaccines, and by vaccine-anxious parents can be summarized as follows:

- Vaccines are not as effective at preventing diseases as health officials claim they are.
- Many side effects—some minor and some serious—are caused by vaccines, and health care professionals understate the number and severity of these side effects.

- We give too many vaccines for too many diseases to children at too young of an age, and we give them too closely together.
- Far too little research has been done to determine the long-term consequences of particular vaccines and their components, the effects of giving multiple vaccines at one time, and the potential susceptibility of some children to side effects from vaccines.
- For-profit pharmaceutical companies exert too much influence on the nation's vaccine policy, and the physicians and public health care officials who shape vaccine policy in the United States work so closely with pharmaceutical companies in the research, manufacture, and sale of vaccines that conflicts of interest seem inevitable.
- Mainstream medical care providers (especially pediatricians) spend too little time discussing the benefits and risks of particular vaccines with parents, too often callously disregard parents' worries or personal beliefs, and respond to concerns in ways that alienate parents.

Health officials generally blame parents' concerns about vaccines on ignorance and a failure to appreciate the danger of communicable diseases. This notion is called into question, however, by poll results that show that concerns about vaccines rise along with rates of educational achievement. The more education a parent has, the more likely he or she will be to question the efficacy and necessity of vaccinations. A 2000 poll found respondents with a high school degree or less were more likely to regard immunization as extremely important than were their more educated peers. Comparing college-educated parents to those with a high school degree or less, college-educated parents were more than twice as likely to refuse to rate immunizations as extremely important in protecting children's health. As a result, almost 17 percent of college graduates chose to opt out of immunizations, while respondents with a high school degree or less opted out at less than 11 percent. A 2007 study of Californian parents' attitudes toward the HPV vaccine had similar results. Nearly 90 percent of the parents who had not finished high school said they were likely to have their daughters vaccinated against HPV, but only about two-thirds of the college graduates would. Precisely the same situation is found in Britain, where middle- and upper-class citizens are less confident about vaccine safety than are working and lower class citizens. This pattern suggests that parents who have higher levels of educational attainment are more likely to question the judgment of medical authorities and public health officials than are their less educated colleagues. Of course, educational attainment is not at all what public health officials mean when they use the term "informed." Instead, it implies willingness by parents to accept the recommendations offered by public health officials and to defer to the authority of their health care providers.[30]

There exists a small group of anti-vaccine parents who avoid all vaccines for their children. Only about 0.3 percent of American children are completely unvaccinated. When asked, nearly half of the parents of unvaccinated children expressed concerns regarding the safety of vaccines. This concern was almost five times more common among parents of completely unvaccinated children than it was among parents of under-vaccinated children. Medical professionals play a smaller role in the decisions made by parents of unvaccinated children than they do in the decisions made by parents of under-vaccinated children. Nearly three-quarters of the parents of unvaccinated children say they made the decision not to vaccinate their children without speaking to their physician, while less than a quarter of the parents of under-vaccinated children reported the same. The parents of unvaccinated children are slightly more commonly white, married, and well educated as compared to the parents of under-vaccinated children, and they tend to have even higher incomes and larger numbers of children than do the parents of under-vaccinated children. In sum, the parents who categorically reject all vaccines seem to share similar demographic attributes with the average vaccine-anxious parent. This should worry public health officials, as it suggests the ease with which vaccine-anxious parents might transform into parents who reject all vaccines for their children. Making the leap from being concerned about vaccines to being an anti-vaccinator does not require a parent to cross cultural or economic boundaries, nor does it require them to adopt a fundamentally different political ideology. All that is needed is an even firmer resolution to allow their anxieties about vaccines to win in their struggle against their pediatricians' and the CDC's recommendations.[31]

American anti-vaccinators and vaccine-anxious parents share notions about the definition of a child's best interest, a reluctance to accept medical advice as universally applicable to all children, and a willingness to go against the establishment (or at least find loopholes that allow their children to avoid being vaccinated). In 2008, the *New York Times* published a story about public health officials' concerns about the increasing numbers of parents who are choosing not to vaccinate their children against certain diseases. It included a picture of three middle-class women, sitting in a nice Californian home, apparently discussing their concerns about vaccines. One of them, Sybil Carlson, has two children, neither of whom has received all of the mandated vaccines. She explained, "When I began to read about vaccines and how they work, I saw medical studies, not given to us by the mainstream media, connecting them with neurological disorders, asthma, and immunology." Having considered her responsibilities both to her children and to the larger public, she said, "I cannot deny that my child can put someone else at risk." Nonetheless, Carlson concluded, "I refuse to sacrifice my children for the greater good." The *New York Times* website received 431 comments on this story in the first twelve hours after it was posted. The intensity of the claims made in support of parents who choose not to vaccinate was matched by the intensity of anger expressed by people who opposed those people.[32]

Carlson and many other parents who have chosen against some or all of the recommended and mandated vaccines for their children are part of an unorganized movement that began two decades ago. It emerged among a limited number of fringe critics of vaccination just as the list of mandatory vaccines was beginning to grow. It established itself in a pre-Internet age through word-of-mouth, and it was advanced by a handful of authors who published with obscure presses and sold their books in venues as culturally diverse as natural health food stores and gun shows. Modern American cultural and ideological notions, not the centuries-old religious opposition to vaccination, form the basis for today's anti-vaccination movement in the United States. Recognizing this fact will allow vaccine proponents to begin from an accurate starting place for considering the source of today's parents' anxieties about vaccines, and to begin responding to the long list of problems that vex the modern American vaccine schedule. There are good reasons to believe that in the near future increasing numbers of vaccine-anxious parents will opt out of some vaccines and that more parents will join the currently tiny percentage of parents who opt out of all vaccines for their children. That means that unless we address the fundamental problems inherent to the modern vaccination schedule, today's vaccine-anxious parents may well become the parents of tomorrow's under-vaccinated and unvaccinated children.

2

Sources of Doubt

It is easy to find claims about the risks posed by particular vaccines—or vaccines generally—to young children. For example, anti-vaccinators often claim that DPT (the vaccine against diphtheria, pertussis, and tetanus) increases a baby's risk of sudden infant death syndrome or deafness and that the varicella vaccine causes sterility in boys. These concerns have at times emerged as a result of published scientific research; for example, in the mid-1990s, researchers hypothesized that administering vaccines to a child at a particular age might increase the chances the child would develop diabetes. Sometimes fears about vaccines follow particular political, national, or ethnic lines, such as the case with the claim circulating within certain African, Muslim, and African American communities that the polio vaccine or the vaccine against hepatitis B caused the AIDS pandemic. Even vaccines given to adults elicit fears of horrible, unintended consequences; it is often claimed that Gulf War Syndrome resulted from the anthrax vaccine that soldiers received. Similarly, there are many reports that the Lyme disease vaccine causes a severe form of arthritis and that the vaccines against tetanus or hepatitis B can cause multiple sclerosis.[1]

Anti-vaccinators' claims have spawned a small industry devoted to publishing their books and pamphlets. For the last two decades, information about vaccines and criticisms of their safety and efficacy were discussed in books from obscure publishers like North Atlantic Books, the New Atlantean Press, Knowledge House, Hatterleigh Press, and Happiness Press. A handful of authors—such as Neil Z. Miller, Randall Neustaedter, and Robert S. Mendelsohn—have published extensive critiques of vaccines, and their books have sold well. The Internet has, of course, been a boon to the anti-vaccination movement, with well-trafficked websites like the National Vaccine Information Center, Vaccination News, Vaccination Liberation, the Vaccine Website, and vaccinationdebate.com. These sources are all readily available to parents with a quick trip to the bookstore or with the stroke of a few keys; they contain an astounding range of authoritative-sounding claims and terrifying anecdotes, capable of worrying any parent, especially one who lacks formal medical training, has preexisting concerns about vaccines, or has a tense relationship with his or her child's pediatrician. Until the late 1990s, anti-vaccination authors' influence was limited to the small number of Americans who adopted "natural" lifestyles, were regular users of alternative medicine, or subscribed to anti-government conspiracy theories. They had little influence on the average American. But now the claims are well known across the social, economic, and political spectrums in the United States, and they animate much of the conversation among parents about their concerns over vaccines.[2]

In this chapter I will examine the origins of the specific beliefs expressed by modern American anti-vaccinators: namely, that vaccines are unsafe, ineffective, untested, and overused. Generally speaking, these notions emerged in the early twentieth century and have evolved alongside the assertions made by the mainstream scientific and medical communities about the incredible power of vaccines to promote public health. What is important here is not to offer a point-by-point critique of the shortcomings of their concerns about vaccines. Responses to criticisms of vaccines are just as easy to find in parenting magazines, professional literature, and on the Internet as are the criticisms themselves. Rather, I want to look specifically at the very different—and originally very fringe—sources from which such claims emanate, and demonstrate how, during the 1990s, they migrated into the mainstream of American thought and coalesced into the set of concerns typically heard from vaccine-anxious parents today.

Our investigation into the wellspring of modern American anti-vaccination sentiment begins with alternative medicine. I will explore its notions generally, recognizing that there are a wide range of unorthodox beliefs, claims, and theories operating under the banner of alternative medicine, some of which contradict one another. Throughout the twentieth century, the most prolific anti-vaccine figures have operated within the confines of alternative medicine. I will briefly discuss the challenge alternative medicine represents to mainstream science and medicine before turning to a close examination of the anti-vaccination sentiment in one particular branch of alternative medicine, chiropractic. Then, I will look at two issues that threw anti-vaccination rhetoric into mainstream conversation: HIV/AIDS and Gulf War Syndrome.[3]

My point in escorting readers through these social and professional movements and for analyzing the basis for their criticism of vaccines is to identify the source of some of today's claims about vaccines. By the turn of the twenty-first century, as the number of mandated childhood vaccines had tripled and a growing number of otherwise mainstream parents grew nervous about vaccines, they had at hand a substantial collection of well-developed critiques of the immunization regime. In this chapter I examine where these now very popular notions originated. Over the subsequent four chapters, I will trace how and why they became so widely known and accepted by many American parents.

Heroes and Cranks

For the past decade, I have taught history of science classes at the University of Puget Sound and at Michigan State University. Both the history of science and the history of medicine are full of stories of heroic protagonists who, despite the dogmas of their day and against tremendous resistance, stood by their guns and were ultimately proven right. Americans especially seem attracted to stories of scientific rebels standing up against established authorities and thereby moving science and medicine forward. From the grave-robbing Vesalius and the heretical Galileo to the supposedly tortured Darwin and the eccentric Einstein, we love seeing history vindicate the scientific David who took on the established Goliath and was later vindicated.

I have often thought I was perhaps doing my students a disservice by teaching them so much about the few scientific rebels who eventually became the leaders of scientific revolutions, especially when the rebels are portrayed as valiantly sticking to their theories despite substantial evidence (and authority) against them. For every scientific rebel who turned out to be right, there are countless others who were just plain wrong. As one historian of science recently noted, "Being in the position of a rebel in the scientific community of one's own time is, of course, one of the potential routes to recognition. To adopt a heretical role in that community is a risky business: it may not ensure fame, and one is very likely to be wrong." I teach my students the virtues of tenacity and dissent, but I avoid giving them the impression that scientific rebels are usually right. The fact is, they are almost always wrong.[4]

Despite my concerns, I recognize the value of the mythology of the lone genius that, through force of conviction and the strength of evidence, could initiate a scientific revolution. The beliefs—whether they are true or not—that scientific claims are constantly subjected to challenge and that any of them could be overthrown at any time is vital to the institutional authority that science enjoys today. In the language of the philosopher of science Karl Popper, for a claim to be considered scientific it must be falsifiable, so every scientific conclusion is necessarily tentative because new evidence can emerge to demonstrate that long-held beliefs are in fact wrong. As we herald the validity of current scientific claims, we point to instances in which previous, long-held scientific beliefs were overturned despite tremendous institutionalized support for them. It is in these instances that the examples of scientific rebels are so valuable.[5]

We can separate the heroes from the cranks when we look backward to see how the current scientific consensus emerged, but it is impossible to do the same thing with a forward-looking perspective. In the middle of a controversy we cannot possibly know whether someone is a budding scientific revolutionary, whose knowledge and tenacity are vital to the advancement of science, or merely a crank. That is precisely the dilemma that vaccine-anxious parents face today when they are confronted with anti-vaccination claims. The prestige and authority of modern science and medicine are of little help in dealing with this issue when it is so easy to find celebrated examples of medical orthodoxy that were so wrong-headed. Remember, the best physicians of the day bled and poisoned George Washington to death as they treated him for a sore throat; nineteenth-century British physicians routinely cut the gums of teething infants, resulting in thousands of deaths from secondary infections. Countless drugs once widely used are now considered too deadly to ever prescribe. There are many currently sanctioned preventative and therapeutic interventions that we will one day find are in fact useless or dangerous, just as there are many approaches advocated by alternative health care providers that will one day be widely accepted within mainstream medicine. Which among the accepted practices are wrong? Who are the budding heroes, and who are the cranks?[6]

Alternative medicine is any healing practice—either preventative or therapeutic—that is not generally accepted by physicians and may not have scientific explanations for how or why it might work. It includes approaches like changes to patients' diets, acupuncture, and megavitamins along with a number of noninvasive therapies—like relaxation techniques, massage, self-help groups, and hypnosis—as well as more mystical treatments like spiritual healing, imagery, and self-prayer. Over the last twenty years, increasing numbers of Americans have turned to alternative medicine to replace or complement mainstream medicine. A 1998 study found the use of alternative therapies increased by over 30 percent during the 1990s, with relaxation techniques, herbal medicine, massage, and chiropractic among the most popular forms.[7]

Fringe critics within the alternative medicine community have the capacity to seriously threaten the social legitimacy of mainstream science and medicine. This is because they simultaneously borrow from the credibility of medical science and caustically critique its foundational ideas. I find it difficult to write about the tension that exists between mainstream science and alternative medicine without employing language from either religion or revolutionary politics. On the one hand, we have the orthodox health care providers who work within the accepted parameters of established authority and represent the accepted standard in preventative and therapeutic medicine. In practice, they follow the dogma of accepted therapeutic and preventative interventions. On the other hand are alternative medicine's rebels, who are branded heretics, prevented entry into orthodox institutions, publicly chastised for their profane worldviews, and labeled a danger to public health.

The impulse to censor unsanctioned approaches is inherent in the notion of a profession, which itself grates against American egalitarian impulses. The mainstream scientific community offers serious challenges to the supposedly democratic and classless ideology of the American political system when it declares its members' claims authoritative and incapable of being adequately challenged by outsiders. Continually since their emergence in the nineteenth century, American physicians, scientists, and public health authorities have struggled to implement their specialized professional knowledge in the context of American egalitarianism and individualism, which itself seems to offer every American the right to be their own expert, especially on matters of personal health. As one colleague recently suggested to me, "Professions have a lot of power, and sometimes they wither under egalitarian impulses. It could be that we are now in one of the egalitarian impulses regarding medicine. With the democratization of information on the web, the authority of medicine has suffered."[8]

Medical authorities worry about how easily anti-vaccinators can spread their message and the lack of oversight that exists in policing their claims. The peer review process is the hallmark of modern science and the method by which scientists reach consensus, challenge one another's conclusions, and limit the influence of outsiders on their work. Peer review, however, is rarely seen among anti-vaccinators, who publish their claims in non-peer-reviewed magazines, newspapers, and paid advertisements. As one critic pointed out, "most of these writings have not been subjected to the critical editorial process undergone by peer-reviewed articles in reputable journals." Anti-vaccinators' claims have therefore not been filtered by modern science's peer-review process.

While peer review is a key tenet in scientific discourse, it is not highly valued in most other venues, certainly not by members of the American alternative health care community. Given that the medical community refuses to endorse most alternative medical providers' methods, there is an obvious circularity in their argument about the importance of the peer review process. They are in effect saying, "We will not accept as legitimate anything that we don't already accept as legitimate." In addition, the cultural and professional norms of many of the groups associated with opposition to vaccination lack the reverence for authority we see among mainstream scientists and physicians. Quite the opposite, they tend to place tremendous value on individuality and self-sufficiency, and they often depict mainstream medicine's resistance to them as a mark of honor.[9]

By the early 1990s, a small cadre of authors had published their criticisms of vaccines in relatively obscure, boutique presses. They cited one another in making "authoritative" statements about the ineffectiveness and dangers of vaccines, and support for their arguments was generally weak. Over the course of the decade, the strength of their arguments and the body of evidence they employed grew substantially. Today, anti-vaccinationists' arguments are elaborate and often persuasive, and they draw extensively—albeit selectively—from mainstream scientific publications. The increasing overlap between orthodox medicine and alternative medicine, the growing sophistication of the arguments, and the divergent worldviews of anti-vaccinationists is nicely illustrated by the growth and popularity of chiropractic in the United States.

Chiropractors

Throughout the twentieth century, chiropractors often served as outspoken critics of the established medical community and especially of physicians' advocacy of vaccines. Chiropractic was founded in the 1890s in Davenport, Iowa, by Daniel David (D. D.) Palmer, who was a practitioner of magnetic therapy. As D. D. Palmer told it, he had been unsuccessful in using magnetic healing techniques to restore the hearing of a man who had lost it seventeen years earlier. However, in the course of the treatment, Palmer noticed an unusually large bump on the back of the man's neck, and he found that one of the man's vertebrae had been "racked from its normal position." He reasoned that if the vertebra was moved back into place, the patient's hearing might return to normal, and after persuading his patient to let him try adjusting the spine, Palmer reported that "soon the man could hear as before."

Exactly how and why this treatment might have worked is unclear, because the cochlear nerve does not pass through the neck. Nonetheless, over the next several years, Palmer developed his notion that disease—or, as he called it, dis-ease—originated in the nervous system and that 95 percent of all illnesses resulted from pinched nerves in the spine. He created a novel method of adjusting patients' spines to allow their bodies to heal themselves and prevent future diseases. In 1897 he began a small school in Davenport, which was subsequently run by his son, Bartlett Joshua (B. J.) Palmer. The younger Palmer was a much more able businessman than his father, and he soon became a dominant and increasingly controversial figure in the development of chiropractic. Under his guidance, the profession grew quickly, and by 1925 his school's enrollment had topped a thousand students. By the 1930s, chiropractic was the largest alternative healing profession in the United States, chiropractors could be licensed in two-thirds of the states, and their average annual incomes were 80 percent of what mainstream physicians earned. From the inception of their profession, chiropractors displayed tremendous individualism and entrepreneurialism; this both resulted from and perpetuates their status as stand-alone providers of health care and contrasts starkly with the mainstream medical system's collectivity and regulation.[10]

For much of the twentieth century, chiropractors held traditional, sometimes even premodern, notions of health and illness. In contrast to mainstream medicine, which was increasingly divorced from religious beliefs, throughout the twentieth century, chiropractors incorporated mysticism and Christian imagery in their descriptions of health, disease, and therapies. They believed disease resulted from a violation of God's natural laws and interruptions of the flow of vital nervous energy, which they called "innate intelligence." Good health required an unobstructed flow of innate intelligence, which was kept moving with simple adjustments of the spinal column that restored health by allowing the body to heal itself. Early chiropractic philosophy was consistent with turn-of-the-century cultural and intellectual assumptions, including a widespread enthusiasm for science and technology, the Midwestern populist movement, and the belief that God was benevolent and ruled the universe through discoverable natural laws. Given the limited capabilities of medicine at the end of the nineteenth century, it was often "more dangerous in sickness to see your doctor than to stay at home and do nothing," as one anthropologist recently noted. B. J. Palmer seriously considered declaring chiropractic a religion, as the laying-on of hands was central to both diagnosis and therapy in chiropractic, and religious language was common in its descriptions and practice. Particularly important to chiropractic was the imagery of persecution at the hands of the established medical professions.[11]

From its inception, chiropractic was in conflict with the increasingly dominant American Medical Association (AMA) and with mainstream physicians generally. The AMA was founded in 1847, when there was little or no licensing for physicians and when medical schools were plentiful, inexpensive, and entirely unregulated. A large number of producers sold a wide variety of patent medicines and nostrums—many of them laden with mercury, opium, or other harmful or addictive substances—directly to consumers. As the germ theory of disease emerged in the mid-nineteenth century, some medical practitioners sought to distinguish their science-based diagnoses and therapies from those offered by those whom they regarded as "quacks." Two years after its founding, the AMA established a board to analyze patent medicines and inform the public about their dangers. The AMA soon developed relationships with emerging pharmaceutical companies, and together they worked to distinguish their legitimate approaches and products from the alternative notions and therapies espoused by unsanctioned manufacturers and practitioners.

By 1901, just as chiropractic was getting started, almost every U.S. state had established a medical board and required a physician to graduate from an AMA-approved medical college in order to be licensed to practice medicine. Five years later, D. D. Palmer became the first of what would eventually be thousands of chiropractors who were arrested and jailed for practicing medicine without a license. Throughout most of the twentieth century, the mainstream medical community aggressively undermined the growth of chiropractic by trying to persuade the American public that chiropractors were not legitimate healthcare providers and by using every available legal means to prevent them from practicing. In 1966, the AMA adopted a policy declaring that the entire medical profession considered chiropractic an "unscientific cult whose practitioners lack the necessary training and background to diagnose and treat human disease," and that therefore "chiropractic constitutes a hazard to rational health care in the United States because of its substandard and unscientific education of its practitioners and their rigid adherence to an irrational, unscientific approach to disease causation."[12]

Until 1978, the AMA regarded it a violation of medical ethics for a licensed physician to have any professional association with a chiropractor or ever to refer a patient to one. In a series of trials that began in 1976, and finally concluded almost a decade and a half later, five chiropractors sued the AMA and ten other healthcare associations claiming they were in violation of the Sherman Antitrust Act for their oppression of chiropractic. The chiropractors eventually won, and the U.S. Court of Appeals affirmed the decision in 1990. As the case was nearing completion, the AMA altered its stance on chiropractic to state that a "physician shall be free to choose whom to serve, with whom to associate, and the environment in which to provide medical services," thus allowing physicians to refer patients to chiropractors without fear of losing their licenses.[13]

By the turn of the twenty-first century, nearly fifty thousand chiropractors were practicing in the United States and smaller numbers in Canada, Australia, and Britain. Their median income approached $100,000 and, according to the U.S. Department of Labor, the "job prospects are expected to be good, especially for those who enter a multi-disciplined practice, consisting of, for example, a chiropractor, physical therapist, and medical doctor." Today, about 11 percent of Americans regularly visit a chiropractor, and more than one-third of insurance companies offer at least partial coverage for chiropractic care. In Canada, where chiropractic care is partially covered in some provinces by the publicly funded health insurance system, one in four Canadians have made use of chiropractic. While chiropractic's popularity has faded from its mid-twentieth-century peak, it is still the third most popular form of alternative medicine in the United States today, behind spiritual healing/prayer and herbal remedies.[14]

As one might expect given chiropractric's long-running struggles with the AMA, its founders' notions about "dis-ease," and the leaders' general rejection of the germ theory of disease, over the last century many chiropractors have been critical about the use of vaccines to improve public health. In his 1909 *The Philosophy of Chiropractic*, B. J. Palmer asserted, "chiropractors have found in every disease that is supposed to be contagious, *a cause in the spine.*" Rather than finding their cause in germs and their prevention with vaccines, Palmer claimed, "There is no contagious disease. . . . There is no infection. . . . There is a cause internal to man that makes of his body in a certain spot, more or less, a breeding ground [for microbes]." As his father had written, "It is the very height of absurdity to strive to 'protect' any person from smallpox or any other malady by inoculating them with a filthy animal poison. . . . No one will ever pollute the blood of any member of my family unless he cares to walk over my dead body to perform such an operation." Vaccination, for the Palmers and their adherents, was at best useless and at worse amounted to poisoning the patient.[15]

Over the twentieth century, as new vaccines emerged, chiropractors honed their arguments against vaccination. By the time the AMA had begun— admittedly begrudgingly—to liberalize its stance toward chiropractic, an entrenched group of chiropractors was expressing serious concerns about the widespread use of vaccines. Today, two principle professional organizations represent chiropractors, the conservative International Chiropractors Association (ICA) and the progressive American Chiropractic Association (ACA). Conservative members of the chiropractic profession tend to avoid working with mainstream physicians and are more likely to see themselves as orthodox descendants of the worldview and methods of the Palmers. In 1990, the ICA adopted a formal statement on vaccines stating that the organization "recognizes that the use of vaccines is not without risk, and is aware of the beneficial consequences of some that have proven to be reasonably safe." Three years later, the more integrationist ACA adopted a policy that accepted that "vaccination has been shown to be a cost-effective and clinically practical public health preventative procedure for certain viral and microbial diseases as demonstrated by the scientific community." Revisions over the next five years to both organizations' statements on vaccines brought them to their current position, which generally accepts that vaccines are a useful tool in maintaining health. It also preserved a space for critics of vaccines by emphasizing that vaccines are "not without risk" and by assertively supporting both an "individual's right to freedom of choice in his/her own health care" and "a conscience clause or waiver in compulsory vaccination laws."[16]

In surveying chiropractors in the United States and in Canada, scholars have uncovered a series of objections against vaccines. Chief among these is the belief that immunizations are simply not effective in preventing disease despite the obvious gains in public health that seemed to accompany their creation and use. For support, they point to the substantial decline in reported cases that occurred shortly before a vaccine was introduced as well as the continued existence of outbreaks in fully vaccinated communities. Diseases, they claim, occur in cyclical patterns, and the perceived effect of the introduction of a vaccine may well simply reflect a natural downturn in the incidence of that particular disease. Some chiropractors also argue that sanitation systems, improved cleanliness, better diet and nutrition, and other public health efforts are responsible for the steep decline in communicable diseases that occurred during the twentieth century. Following this line of argument, they point to disease outbreaks in highly vaccinated communities as evidence that vaccines are simply not capable of ridding populations of communicable diseases.

Chiropractors' emphasis on natural methods to enhance their patients' health sometimes leads them to argue that childhood diseases ultimately serve a protective purpose and that the use of vaccines undermines that benefit. They claim that it is beneficial for a child to contract diseases like measles or chickenpox because, as one chiropractor argued, they "'prime' and mature a child's immune system" by teaching "a child's immune system to fight off an infection on its own." Lacking this immunological training, they argue, a vaccinated child is "susceptible to a more serious complication later in life." Many communicable diseases are much less serious when contracted earlier in life, which is often offered as evidence that weathering childhood diseases, rather than avoiding them, is the superior method for acquiring good health.[17]

Chiropractors who are critical of vaccines also emphasize the potential side effects of vaccines. In addition to the adverse reactions described in the mainstream medical literature, they assert that a myriad of more recently described diseases find their origin with the widespread implementation of immunization programs. As one conservative chiropractor argued in a 1999 letter to the editor in Ontario's *Burlington Post*, "One of the concerns is there has been a drastic increase in the numbers of autoimmune diseases seen: everything from diabetes to asthma, autism, Crohn's disease, AIDS, cancer, etc." In making these claims, they highlight whatever disagreement might exist among mainstream medical providers regarding vaccine policy and emphasize that no research—or, at the very least, insufficient research—has been done to determine the long-term effects of immunization. In this regard, they assert that vaccination programs are essentially no more than human experimentations conducted on a massive scale.[18]

Finally, drawing on their long history of battling the AMA and arguing that mainstream medical authorities and pharmaceutical companies have had undue influence on Americans' health, they assert that American immunization policy is governed by the "medical-pharmaceutical complex" and motivated by greed. Chiropractic literature makes frequent inferences about "conflicts of interest, bribery, and scientific fraud. Suggestions of government conspiracies, distortions of truth, and cover-ups abound." Some chiropractors argue this activity is sanctioned by government officials who inappropriately compel citizens to receive vaccines. They point to the role of industry in establishing national vaccine policy. Chiropractors who oppose vaccines assert that the top scientific and medical officials who serve on advisory boards have committed serious breaches of medical ethics because of the conflicts of interest that result from their involvement in the research and manufacturing of vaccines and the financial windfalls that result from a new vaccine being included among states' mandated immunizations.[19]

A 2002 survey of students enrolled in the Canadian Memorial Chiropractic College (CMCC), which trains about 80 percent of the nation's chiropractors, found that about half reported they were generally supportive of vaccination efforts. This was good news for both mainstream physicians in Canada as well as for the chiropractic college, because the school's curriculum supported vaccines. Most students believed that the college's core lectures presented vaccination either positively or at least neutrally. The bad news, however, was that students became increasingly critical of vaccines as they progressed through their four years of education at CMCC. Among first-year students, over 60 percent reported that in general they agreed with vaccination. By the time they had become fourth-year students, less than 40 percent did. In describing the source of this dramatic drop in students' support for vaccines as they progressed through their four years of chiropractic education, the survey's authors explained that while the college's official curriculum was strongly supportive of vaccines, "Invited lecturers speaking in informal settings were perceived by most students as presenting vaccination negatively." The researchers explained, "Within the chiropractic profession, ultraconservative practitioners, known as 'straight,' 'principled,' 'on-purpose,' or 'purpose-straight' chiropractors, maintain a literal interpretation of the theories of D. D. Palmer, the founder of chiropractic."

While the view of the "straight" members of the profession have very little influence over the CMCC's curriculum, student groups, clubs and invited speakers bring their conservative views to campus. In the invited commentary that appeared along with the report of the survey's findings, two employees of the Centers for Disease Control and Prevention (CDC) discussed the "unsettling trend during the professional education of chiropractic students." "In light of the growing prevalence of chiropractic care in Canada and elsewhere," they warned readers, "there is a risk that these attitudes will be passed on to patients." Given that the CMCC's curriculum was already supportive of vaccines and that it appeared that anti-vaccination sentiment was presented to students in extracurricular activities over which the school could exert only limited control, the commentators argued the best course of action would be to further integrate chiropractic with mainstream medicine. The nation's largest medical school, the University of Toronto, was located close to CMCC, and the commentators suggested their proximity would allow students at the two schools to work together in promoting vaccination programs. It might be, they asserted, "an ideal model for encouraging medical and chiropractic students to work together and to learn from each other. To our knowledge, such collaboration has not been formally attempted."[20]

In the history of chiropractic and its attitudes toward vaccination, two issues are directly relevant to the modern American vaccine controversy. First, many of the concerns expressed by today's vaccine-anxious parents are found in the assertions made by conservative chiropractors throughout the twentieth century:

- It is wrong to force people to vaccinate themselves and their children against their will.
- Vaccines are ineffective at preventing diseases.
- Vaccines are unnatural interventions not in the long-term best interests of an individual's health and wellbeing.
- Vaccines have serious and unavoidable side effects.
- There is insufficient research into the efficacy and safety of vaccines both individually and collectively.
- The modern vaccine regime is the product of the greed and authoritarianism of the medical community acting in concert with large, wealthy pharmaceutical companies.

Today, many of these aspersions are cast against individual vaccines rather than against vaccines in general, as the "straight" chiropractors have been doing for the last century. For example, anti-vaccinators frequently criticize the chickenpox vaccine as unnecessary (because it protects against a very minor childhood illness) and ineffective (because of recent research that suggests its efficacy fades after five years). Likewise the human papillomavirus (HPV) vaccine has come under heavy criticism because of how quickly it was researched, approved, and sent to market, the limited amount of research done to demonstrate its efficacy and safety, and the manner in which Merck lobbied to have it included among states' mandated vaccines.

The second lesson we can draw from chiropractors' resistance to vaccines can be found in how effective mainstream medicine was in swaying chiropractors over to supporting, or at least not overtly undermining, vaccines by working collaboratively and being respectful of their beliefs and norms. The recent willingness of the AMA—albeit under threat of legal action from the federal government—to remove sanctions against the licensed physicians who wanted to collaborate with chiropractors, and calls in medical journals for "medical and chiropractic students to work together," suggest ways to minimize the effects of anti-vaccination sentiment among some chiropractors. There is obviously much to be gained in terms of minimizing the impact of the longstanding anti-vaccine undercurrent among chiropractors by bringing willing chiropractors into the fold of mainstream medicine. Certainly, there are some conservative chiropractors whose views and recommendations will not be swayed from their ardent anti-vaccine positions because, as one recent author asserted, "their views on immunization may not be based on evidence, or open to scientific scrutiny, but rather on the demands of their faith/belief system/philosophy." However, conservative views exist among a relatively small number of chiropractic (and chiropractic-associated) authors who continue to disseminate anti-vaccination views. But nearly thirty-five million Americans regularly visit a chiropractor, and there is a great deal that can be done in cooperation with progressive chiropractors who see themselves working in collaboration with mainstream medical therapies. This can happen only if scientists and physicians are willing to abandon the combative and authoritarian stance they took toward chiropractic and other forms of alternative medicine throughout the twentieth century. As patients adopt new branches of alternative medicine, mainstream medical providers would be wise to remember the example of chiropractic and take care to avoid placing their patients in the position of having to choose between their two competing worldviews. Otherwise, every parent who chooses an alternative therapy means potentially one more undervaccinated child.[21]

By the turn of the twenty-first century, conservative opposition to vaccines continued among some chiropractors and emerged in the alternative medical community. Anti-vaccinators' claims and their influence were limited to the relatively small number of Americans who were consumers of alternative medical therapies. It would take a couple of dramatic medical mysteries to help bring anti-vaccination concerns into the mainstream in the 1990s: AIDS and Gulf War Syndrome.

AIDS and the Polio Vaccine

The mysterious ailment that came to be known as AIDS first came to the attention of public health authorities in 1981 when the CDC recorded a cluster of cases of *Pneumocystis carini* pneumonia, a rare, opportunistic lung infection that is sometimes found in people with compromised immune systems, as well as clusters of cases of Kaposi's sarcoma, skin tumors caused by the human herpesvirus 8. The first cases occurred among a group of gay men in Los Angeles and New York, and the officials at the CDC struggled to determine their root cause. The American press soon began reporting on what it called gay-related immune deficiency (GRID), but the CDC eventually realized that anyone, regardless of sexual orientation, could be affected. In 1982 officials began referring to the ailment as acquired immunodeficiency syndrome (AIDS), and a year later, two different research groups reported in the journal *Science* that they had determined that AIDS was caused by a novel retrovirus that was officially named the human immunodeficiency virus (HIV). By that time, other researchers had discovered similar ailments among captive monkeys, which led to the determination that HIV had originated with the simian immunodeficiency viruses (SIV). Variations of SIV are frequently found in dozens of different species of African primates, but only two particular variations of it appear to be responsible for the strains of HIV found in humans: SIVsmm from sooty mangabeys are believed to be the source of HIV-1, and SIVcpz from chimpanzees are believed to be the origin of HIV-2.

By the late 1980s, researchers had determined that AIDS was caused by HIV, which had somehow crossed the species barrier from monkeys into humans sometime in the first half of the twentieth century. The most common explanation for the first human infection with HIV is the natural transfer hypothesis, which is sometimes called the cut-hunter theory or the monkey-bite hypothesis. It supposes that the transference of SIV into humans came when someone came in contact with SIV while hunting, butchering, or eating an infected chimpanzee and subsequently developed HIV-1. Researchers have offered a similar explanation for the transference of SIVsmm into humans and its development into HIV-2. Today, nearly three decades after AIDS first came to the attention of American health officials, the natural transfer hypothesis is the most widely accepted explanation for how SIV leapt the species barrier from monkeys to humans, became HIV, and initiated the worldwide AIDS pandemic. It is not, however, the only theory.[22]

While the mainstream scientific community had come to nearly universal agreement on the origins of HIV/AIDS, a contradictory theory explaining its emergence developed within the alternative medicine community that implicated the polio vaccine as the source of the AIDS epidemic. In 1987, on the radio show "Natural Living," which was broadcast on WABC in New York, the show's host, Gary Null, interviewed Eva Lee Snead, a holistic health advocate and a longtime opponent of vaccination. Snead appears to be the first to have suggested a connection between the polio vaccine and the emergence of AIDS. Louis Pascal, an independent scholar, heard the radio show and wrote a long article that drew from medical journals published in the 1950s and 1960s to conclude that a particular form of the polio vaccine widely administered in the Belgian Congo in the late 1950s was the likely source of the original HIV infections. He submitted the article to several scientific journals, including the *Lancet, Nature, New Scientist,* and the *Journal of Medical Ethics,* and all of them rejected it. Pascal asserts their rejection of the paper was part of the medical community's "clear attempts at whitewash," but for his part, the editor of the *Journal of Medical Ethics* acknowledged the importance of Pascal's paper and wrote an editorial to publicize the paper's eventual publication on the Internet. In it, the editor explained he had asked Pascal to cut the paper down from its overwhelmingly large nineteen thousand words to less than three thousand five hundred and to add some material to it that would "consider the ethical issues that would be raised by publication of material that might well dissuade large numbers of people from having their infants vaccinated against polio and perhaps against other infections."[23]

At about the same time, Blaine Elswood, a San Francisco AIDS activist, had developed a similar hypothesis asserting a link between the mass polio vaccinations in Africa and the emergence of HIV and AIDS. Elswood had helped to found a number of "guerrilla clinics" that conducted research and provided alternative treatments for people suffering with AIDS. In 1991, he mailed a stack of scientific articles to Tom Curtis, an investigative journalist in Houston, Texas, along with a note that said, "Here's a bombshell story just waiting for an investigative reporter." The following year Curtis published "The Origin of AIDS" in *Rolling Stone,* and the competing theory of the origin of AIDS leaped from the relatively insulated alternative health community into mainstream conversation.[24]

Curtis's article, written in the lucid *Rolling Stone* investigative style, laid out the argument that HIV had been accidentally introduced into humans during the massive vaccination campaigns against polio with the oral polio vaccine (OPV) in Africa in the 1950s and 1960s. Several competing research groups had been working to develop easily administrable, safe, and effective vaccines against polio. In 1954, Hilary Koprowski reported that his team had developed the CHAT vaccine, named after Charleton, the child who donated the sample that ultimately led to the vaccine's development. The CHAT polio vaccine was licensed by the U.S. Food and Drug Administration and endorsed for widespread use by the World Health Organization. It was manufactured by growing the virus in a tissue culture—usually fresh monkey kidneys—then inactivating it with formaldehyde. The resulting vaccine was administered by squirting a small amount of it in patients' mouths, which meant that large numbers of people could be quickly vaccinated with the oral polio vaccine.

When the polio vaccine campaigns began in the 1950s, there were relatively few safety standards governing research on and manufacture of vaccines, so a number of unidentified monkey viruses found their way into the vaccines, at least some of which proved deadly to researchers and employees of vaccine manufacturers. For example, the so-called monkey B virus—now known as *Cercopithecine herpesvirus* 1—killed several of the caretakers who worked with Rhesus monkeys imported from India. Other vaccines exposed the people who were inoculated with them to viruses that may or may not have caused them health problems. Between 1954 and 1963 tens of millions of people were exposed to SV40, a virus that infected the kidneys of

Asian Rhesus monkeys, when it contaminated polio vaccines. The OPV AIDS hypothesis, as it has come to be called, asserts that tissues from SIV infected monkeys were used to produce the CHAT polio vaccine, which was then given to at least 325,000 people in the parts of Africa that are now the Democratic Republic of the Congo, Rwanda, and Burundi. That same region has been determined to be the origin of AIDS, and advocates of the OPV AIDS hypothesis assert that the slack safety standards used in the manufacture of the OPV allowed one or more versions of SIV, for which there was no screening prior to its discovery in 1985, to find its way into some of the vaccines, which then led to the introduction of HIV into humans. In 1993, a year after Curtis's article was published, Koprowski sued both *Rolling Stone* and Tom Curtis for defamation. Just before Koprowski had been scheduled to undergo deposition, his lawyers settled with *Rolling Stone* for one dollar and a promise to publish a statement. The lawsuit effectively shut down most media discussion on the OPV AIDS hypothesis, as Curtis was unable to pursue the subject further without adding additional evidence to the case against him.[25]

The scientific and medical communities have been steadfast in rejecting the claims that are associated with the OPV AIDS hypothesis. Beginning with Koprowski's lawsuit against *Rolling Stone* and the $300,000 he spent on lawyers, and extending into the tremendous amount of ink spilled in scientific and medical journals refuting the hypothesis, the mainstream scientific and medical establishments have made clear that the OPV AIDS hypothesis is not part of the orthodox interpretation of the origin and spread of HIV/AIDS. Curtis's article initially generated substantial media coverage in reports by Reuters, UPI, CNN's *Larry King Live,* and *Time* magazine. In response, the CDC issued an official statement asserting that the "weight of scientific evidence does not support this idea." In the fall of 1992, six months after the *Rolling Stone* article, an independent committee of scientists reported that the chance that the OPV AIDS hypothesis was true was "extremely low," but that nonetheless serious efforts ought to be made to stop using monkey kidneys for culturing polio vaccines. Despite the substantial investigative work conducted by Tom Curtis, Blaine Elsworth, and Louis Pascal, none of them were contacted by the committee during the course of its inquiry.[26]

The OPV AIDS hypothesis reached its fullest expression in the 2000 book *The River: A Journey to the Source of HIV and AIDS* by Edward Hooper, a British journalist. Hooper first encountered the OPV AIDS hypothesis when he read Curtis's 1992 *Rolling Stone* article, and his nearly twelve-hundred-page tome was the product of seven years' research in the United States, Europe, and Africa. It begins with a brief description of the nineteenth-century debate over the official origin of the Nile River, a concept that he uses throughout the book as a metaphor for the debate over the origin of AIDS. Both debates involved Western authorities and their influence over the African continent, and both the source of the Nile and the source of AIDS, according to Hooper, were originally misidentified. The book is compellingly written, and Hooper employs a variety of rhetorical tools to help the reader keep track of over two hundred and fifty characters as well as water metaphors and allusions to prominent events in medical history like John Snow's removal of the Broad Street pump handle, which helped end the 1854 London cholera epidemic and gave birth to modern epidemiology. In brief, Hooper asserts that an experimental oral polio vaccine was the route by which SIV made the leap into humans and evolved into HIV. He avoids taking an accusatory tone, and instead emphasizes the need for the scientific and medical communities to aggressively pursue and test the OPV AIDS hypothesis. Today, Hooper continues to advance the argument through his website, aidsorgins .com, which offers many documents and publications related to the debate of the OPV AIDS hypothesis. *The River* was widely reviewed in the popular press in both the United States and in Britain, and many of the reviews were highly positive.[27]

Hooper's epic book, with its voluminous detail, made an excellent target for scientists, public health officials, and physicians who sought to undermine the OPV AIDS hypothesis. William Donald Hamilton, an eminent British evolutionary biologist, developed a professional interest in Hooper's work, and the two became friends and collaborators when Hamilton agreed to write what Hooper called "a surprisingly hard-hitting foreword" to *The River*. Given Hamilton's scientific prestige and his position as a Royal Society research professor, his involvement in *The River* led to a special two-day Royal Society conference on the origins of HIV in September of 2000. The OPV AIDS hypothesis took center stage when researchers revealed that "tests of old samples of the vaccine provided no supporting evidence" for it. As the journal *Science* reported, Hooper "endured a verbal battering himself from several prominent scientists. But Hooper, unbowed, got in plenty of jabs of his own." In the end, Hooper and his advocates appeared unshaken in their views on the OPV AIDS hypothesis, as did their opponents. Over the next four years, several new studies emerged that further discredited the hypothesis that HIV

was started or spread through the oral polio vaccine. By 2001, most researchers believed—and continue to believe—that HIV diverged from SIV and established itself in humans sometime in the first third of the twentieth century, predating the oral polio vaccine and making the OPV AIDS hypothesis
incorrect. The natural transfer hypothesis, not the OPV AIDS hypothesis, is
the officially accepted assumption of how SIV made its way into humans and
evolved into HIV.[28]

In the 1990s, there emerged a handful of other propositions linking HIV
and AIDS to vaccines. The same month that Curtis published his article in
Rolling Stone, Walter S. Kyle, an attorney who specialized in vaccine injury
law, published an opinion piece in the *Lancet*. He argued that HIV-related
retroviruses infected some lots of the polio vaccine and that off-label use of
OPV in the 1970s to treat homosexuals who suffered recurrent herpes infections had introduced HIV into a population of gay men in the United States.
Other authors pointed to the disposable syringes used to inoculate people
and suggested that in resource-starved Africa, healthcare workers might have
unknowingly spread the HIV infection—however it was first started—by re-
using unsterile needles. These claims, like the OPV AIDS hypothesis, placed
blame on the public health community for spreading HIV and stirred
concern among some people who already worried about mass vaccination
programs.[29]

Conspiracy theories were common amid speculations about the origin of
HIV and AIDS, especially theories alleging that HIV was manmade and was
intentionally introduced into humans by way of a vaccine. The notion appears to have originated with Jakob Segal, a biology professor at Humboldt
University in former East Germany who was later accused of being a Soviet
disinformation agent. In 1986, he published a pamphlet in which he claimed
that scientists at a military lab in Fort Detrick, Maryland, manufactured HIV
by synthesizing a retrovirus that causes leukemia from a sheep virus and
then injected it into prisoners. The claim that HIV/AIDS was the product of
the U.S. military's work with a sheep virus was popular in the Soviet Union
in the 1980s and appeared in a nonscientific journal article written by a Soviet
official, Valentin Zapevalov. In the United States, Boyd Graves, a lawyer who
tested positive for HIV, has claimed that the virus was created when the "U.S.
Special Virus Program" altered a sheep virus and, with help from the pharmaceutical company Merck, added it to an experimental hepatitis B vaccine
and gave it to gay men and blacks in New York City and San Francisco. In

1994, Gary Glum, a Los Angeles lawyer and advocate of an herbal cancer cure, published *Full Disclosure* in which he asserted that scientists at the Cold Spring Harbor Laboratory in New York engineered HIV to wipe out the world's black population, and that the World Health Organization intentionally spread it under cover of its smallpox eradication efforts.

Among the most prolific of the authors who have advanced claims about a link between HIV/AIDS and vaccines is Alan Cantwell Jr., a retired dermatologist who published several books in the 1980s and 1990s alleging that HIV is the result of a government-sponsored hepatitis B vaccine experiment that used gay men in New York and California as guinea pigs. Similarly, Neil Z. Miller devoted a chapter of his *Immunization Theory vs. Reality: Exposé on Vaccinations* to the links between HIV/AIDS and vaccination. In the chapter "Genocide," Miller asserted, "Researchers are considering at least two plausible lines of inquiry—high probability links—between vaccines and AIDS." The first is a brief restatement of the OPV AIDS hypothesis followed by a description of a civil tort claim filed in 1994 by the mother of a twelve-year-old girl who had tested HIV-positive, who alleged that her daughter had contracted HIV when she was given the live virus oral polio vaccine in 1992. The second of the so-called "high probability links," according to Miller, was that HIV and AIDS were the result of a biological warfare experiment conducted by the United States government in which animal viruses were "synthetically altered and added to the smallpox vaccine," which was then "tested on millions of unsuspecting Central Africans during the 1970s." Miller presents little evidence and his arguments are undeveloped, but some of his claims coincide with the much more thoroughly researched and argued work done by Curtis and Hooper.[30]

The conspiracy theories that emerged around the mysterious origin of AIDS spread quickly and became deeply rooted in the African American community. A 2005 survey found that half of the five hundred African Americans surveyed said they believed that HIV was a man-made virus, while a quarter of them believed it was created in a government laboratory, and approximately 12 percent believed it was intentionally created and spread by the Central Intelligence Agency. The survey also found that slightly more than half believed that the government was withholding a cure for AIDS from the poor. Jeremiah Wright, the former pastor of the Trinity United Church of Christ, a megachurch in Chicago with eight thousand five hundred members, and the former pastor of President Barack Obama, also advanced the notion that HIV and AIDS were man-made diseases. In 2008, ABC News reviewed dozens of Wright's sermons, excerpted parts of them, and opened him and then-candidate Obama to intense media scrutiny. Among the excerpts was one in which Wright said, "the U.S. government invented AIDS to destroy people of color." For his part, Obama distanced himself from Wright's remarks about the treatment of minorities in the United States and categorically rejected his claim that the United States government invented AIDS to destroy black people.[31]

Conspiracy theories about the origin of AIDS and potential links to the polio vaccine circulated outside the United States as well. For example, shortly before the Kenyan environmentalist Wangari Maathai received the Nobel Peace Prize, she told participants at an AIDS workshop in Nyeri, Kenya, "AIDS is not a curse from God to Africans or the black people. It is a tool to control them designed by some evil-minded scientists." The day after she was named the 2004 Nobel Peace Prize laureate, she was quoted as saying, "I may not be able to say who developed the virus, but it was meant to wipe out the black race."

Concerns about the safety of the polio vaccine have taken a serious toll on public health officials' efforts to eradicate polio. In 1988, health authorities set the year 2000 as a target year for their goal. They failed to meet it, but by 2003 they had successfully rid it from all but six countries. That same year, Muslim imams and local politicians in Nigeria began spreading rumors that the polio vaccine could make women sterile, contained pork products, or could transmit AIDS. These claims were repeated throughout much of the Muslim world, and by 2005 the disease had spread back into an additional sixteen countries.[32]

Today, the scientific community is nearly unanimous in its belief that SIV found its way into humans and initiated the HIV/AIDS pandemic sometime between the early nineteenth century and the mid-twentieth century. The most recent research suggests that HIV simmered in relatively small pockets of the human population for a time, before social, political, and cultural developments led it to explode near the end of the twentieth century. One frequently invoked explanation is that urban migration and increasing sexual contact explain HIV's transformation into a pandemic disease. Another explanation, perhaps the most widely held among scientists today, asserts that the explosive spread of HIV was due to the introduction into Africa of millions of inexpensive, mass-produced syringes in the 1950s that accompanied campaigns to stamp out syphilis, malaria, smallpox, and polio. Many traditional healers used and reused the syringes in the production of herbal remedies, and African families owned and used the syringes without properly sterilizing them. This explanation accepts that medical products might have played an important role in spreading HIV while exonerating Western medical professionals from direct responsibility.[33]

As we consider modern American concerns about vaccines and the claim that the global campaign against polio initiated today's global AIDS epidemic, there are three important issues that emerge. First, the alternative medical community served as an incubator for theories about the origins of HIV/AIDS and especially for the OPV AIDS hypothesis. The allegation that AIDS was a manmade pandemic that was caused by carelessness in the manufacture of the CHAT polio vaccine was first made by Eva Snead on Gary Null's radio program in 1987. Null has made a career of offering expert guidance to anyone interested in pursuing lifestyles and therapies outside of mainstream medicine. He bills himself as "America's Leading Health and Nutrition Expert" and offers "an on-air health forum" on radio stations from coast to coast. He is also a prolific author who has published on topics closely associated with contemporary alternative medicine and has produced a documentary movie, *The Vaccine Nation*, that "challenges the basic health claims by government health agencies and pharmaceutical firms that vaccines are perfectly safe." His views on vaccines are clear: they are neither safe nor effective. In a recent statement on the influenza vaccine, for example, Null stated, "The American public has every reason to be suspicious over our health officials' vaccination claims and to hold them in distrust and even contempt." By the 1990s, as modern American anti-vaccination sentiment was emerging, the OPV AIDS hypothesis was well established in the fertile ground offered by the alternative medical community. Given the right conditions, it leaped into the mainstream. Clearly, one of the necessary conditions for the story to be picked up by U.S. parents was the emergence of a more general concern by Americans about vaccines. Health officials need to address the vaccine anxieties that have developed among the average American parent, not the fringe claims that provide the language for these concerns to be expressed.[34]

Second, we see in the mainstream scientific and medical communities' responses evident concern that the OPV AIDS hypothesis might diminish the public's confidence in the polio vaccine specifically and in vaccines generally. Even before Curtis published his article in *Rolling Stone*, the editor of the

Journal of Medical Ethics asked Pascal to consider ethical issues that might arise from his work if it discouraged large numbers of people from vaccinating their children against polio or other diseases. Shortly after Hooper published *The River*, the editor of the journal *Nature* called for a truce in the debate over the OPV AIDS hypothesis, because he feared that the "public confidence in vaccines" could be undermined if the debate continued. In his review of Hooper's *The River* in the journal *Nature*, John P. Moore of the Aaron Diamond AIDS Research Center at Rockefeller University compared the OPV AIDS hypothesis to conspiracy theories about the assassination of President John F. Kennedy and concluded, "My biggest concern over this book is that it could reinforce public distrust of science and scientists." In dismissing Hooper's claims in *The River*, Koprowski warned that Hooper's "allegations were undermining polio vaccination efforts in Africa," pointing out that the Catholic Church in Kenya was advising parents not to have their children vaccinated because of the dangers of contamination. In 2000, when the tests of the vaccine samples of CHAT failed to show any trace of SIV or HIV, officials at the Wistar Institute announced that the findings would "soothe public concern over the safety of vaccines, which had been raised by the allegations." The acting director stated, "We trust that these results will put to rest any remaining concerns of a link between Wistar-produced oral polio vaccine and AIDS. The findings should also serve to restore public confidence in the production and administration of vaccines."[35]

Even years after the scientific and medical communities rejected the OPV AIDS hypothesis, researchers and physicians continued to hammer away at it by publishing even more refutations of it. In doing so, researchers and health officials have been clear that they are motivated by a sincere concern about the public's confidence in vaccines. For example, in 2004 researchers at the University of Arizona discovered a new strain of SIV in chimpanzees and concluded that it demonstrated that chimps in that area could not have been the source of HIV. They found that the strain circulating in the species of chimpanzees used to produce the OPV was "phylogenetically distinct from all strains of HIV-1, providing direct evidence that these chimpanzees were not the source of the human AIDS pandemic." In their article they asserted that, in light of current fears in some parts of the world about the safety of polio vaccines, "our clear-cut evidence against one of the key sources of concern is timely."[36]

Finally, the allegation that carelessness in the manufacture of the polio vaccine allowed SIV to cross the species barrier from monkeys into humans powerfully supports current concerns about the safety of today's vaccines as well as allegations that pharmaceutical companies are not sufficiently cautious in researching and producing new vaccines. In the issue of *Rolling Stone* that followed Curtis's 1992 article, one reader asked, "How can researchers be sure other vaccines, or medicines, are not contaminated with other as yet unknown retroviruses?" The scientific community has not been blind to the fact that the OPV AIDS hypothesis, whether it was true or not, revealed an astonishing lack of care in the manufacture of the oral polio vaccine. This realization led to calls, often made in the midst of arguments against the OPV AIDS hypothesis, to improve safety standards by no longer using tissues taken from recently killed animals and instead using cells that have been cultured in the laboratory and can more easily be screened for contamination.[37]

The public and professional debates over the OPV AIDS hypothesis imported some of the alternative medical community's concerns about the unintended consequences of vaccines into mainstream discussion. At the same time, another medical mystery emerged that pressed these concerns even deeper into the public's consciousness. Claims that vaccines were somehow involved in the symptoms associated with Gulf War Syndrome brought vaccine anxieties to an entirely different segment of the American public and furthered the public's concerns about vaccines generally.

Vaccines and Gulf War Syndrome

By the end of the Persian Gulf War in 1991, Coalition forces had sent nearly a million personnel to the conflict. Officially, the United States was joined by thirty-six nations during the war, plus three additional nations who provided financial or logistical aid but did not lend military assistance. American forces did the vast majority of the fighting, with the French, British, Canadians, Danes, and Australians also committing some troops to the effort. In total, almost 700,000 American soldiers were sent to the region, while the British sent 43,000 troops; the French sent 18,000; the Canadians provided four ships, a squadron of fighter jets, and a military hospital; the Australians contributed a small number of ships and aircraft; and the Danes sent nearly 1,000 military personnel to assist in peacekeeping and cleanup after the war ended.[38]

Death rates for U.S. soldiers were very low, with only 372 total deaths among American military personnel, over half of them from accidents. The low death rate can be credited to the tremendous preparation undertaken in the months leading up to the conflict and to intelligence efforts that pinpointed most of Iraq's military assets. Intelligence reports indicated that Iraq had successfully weaponized anthrax, botulinum, and aflatoxin, so preparedness efforts included vaccinating troops to protect them against attacks with missiles that carried warheads packed with biological weapons.[39]

Throughout the so-called first Gulf War, the American presence in the Gulf in the 1990s, into the start of what has been called the second Gulf War (or the Iraq War), and during the American occupation of Iraq, soldiers and some civilian personnel received mandatory vaccines against anthrax, plague, typhoid, and botulinum. In 2002, federal courts rejected several challenges to the military's forced vaccinations, but in 2004 the U.S. District Court of the District of Columbia decided that the military could not require soldiers to receive anthrax vaccinations, although it could vaccinate the soldiers who volunteered for the shots. After the ruling, only about half of the troops who were offered the shot accepted it. In October 2006 the Pentagon announced that it would resume requiring anthrax vaccines for troops and civilian personnel serving in Afghanistan, Iraq, and South Korea because, according to William Winkenwerder Jr., the assistant secretary of defense for health affairs, the threat of an anthrax attack was "very real." The military restarted the mandatory vaccination program following a final order from the U.S. Food and Drug Administration that declared the anthrax vaccine safe and effective in preventing anthrax.[40]

Soon after American troops began returning home from Iraq, reports of mysterious illnesses emerged. Symptoms varied, but they generally included fatigue, headaches and memory problems, muscle and joint pain, and digestive problems, and they seemed to affect about a third of the men and women who served in the first Gulf War. Perhaps even more disturbing, problems were also showing up in the children produced by Gulf War veterans. Men who served in the Gulf War were 1.8 times more likely than their nonveteran counterparts to have children with birth defects and women were 2.8 times more likely. Additional research found that British veterans were suffering from similar ailments at about the same rates as their U.S. counterparts, while Australian, Canadian, and Danish troops showed some symptoms as well, but at much lower rates. Initially, the U.S. military and the Central Intelligence Agency concluded the illnesses were the result of the inadvertent destruction of an Iraqi ammunition dump at Khamisiyah that had been stocked with chemical weapons. But there were a number of lingering problems with that conclusion; most notably, the symptoms that the veterans were having did not correlate to exposure to chemical weapons.[41]

Beginning in 1998, the U.S. Congress ordered a series of reports—nine in total—from the National Academies of Science's Institute of Medicine (IOM) to help uncover the cause or causes of the ailments that were afflicting so many Gulf War veterans. In addition to the usual physical and mental challenges personnel faced in a war zone, soldiers in the Gulf War were exposed to a combination of potential health hazards unlike anything experienced in prior conflicts. These including vaccines against biological weapons, prophylactic medicines to protect against nerve agents, exposure to depleted uranium munitions, nerve agents released when Iraqi weapons depots were destroyed, terrible environmental conditions created by burning oil wells, and the widespread use of toxic pesticides. The committee found that the emerging research suggested that psychiatric illnesses caused by stress did not adequately explain the ailments, and they looked to other environmental factors for a source. Finally, in 2010, almost two decades after the Gulf War began, the committee of the IOM that was charged with investigating soldiers' complaints of illness announced that Gulf War Syndrome was indeed "real" and stated that it "may reflect interactions between environmental exposures and genes, such that genetics predisposed many troops to illness." The next line of research on the issue, the committee concluded, should focus on the question of genetics.[42]

Almost as soon as symptoms appeared and the notion emerged that there might be a medical syndrome affecting the soldiers who had served in the Gulf War, vaccine opponents linked the ailments directly to the vaccines American soldiers received before and during the war, especially the anthrax vaccine. In his 1996 book *Immunization Theory vs. Reality: Exposé on Vaccinations*, Neil Miller argued incorrectly that the broad range of symptoms associated with what was being called "Gulf War Syndrome" were all limited to U.S. soldiers, who were also the only ones who had received experimental vaccinations against botulism and anthrax as well as the prophylactic anti-nerve agent drug pyridostigmine. Miller asserted that the soldiers' forced vaccinations represented human experimentation done without adequate disclosure by the medical and military authorities. He concluded emphatically, "Despite vaccine propaganda claiming the shots are safe and effective, consumers should beware of these potentially dangerous drugs and the unscrupulous forces pressing for our compliance. We are not their human guinea pigs!"[43]

In 2003, Gary Null—who had introduced the world to the OPV AIDS hypothesis when he interviewed Eva Snead on his radio show in 1987—joined the public discussion about vaccines and the military when he published *Germs, Biological Warfare, Vaccinations: What You Need to Know.* Null's book was marketed in the aftermath of the 9/11 terrorist attacks and the unsolved anthrax attacks that killed five people and infected seventeen others. Bioterrorism was a significant concern to Americans, who were gearing up for an invasion of Iraq based on the claim that Saddam Hussein had both biological weapons and weapons of mass destruction. (The eventual suspect in the 2001 mailing of packages containing anthrax spores, Bruce Edwards Ivins, was a scientist who worked at the U.S. government's biodefense lab at Fort Detrick in Frederick, Maryland, the same lab that AIDS conspiracy proponents like Jakob Segal claimed produced HIV. Ivins died of an overdose of acetaminophen in an apparent suicide after learning that charges would be filed against him.) Null asserted that, in the rush to prepare for the war and motivated by tremendous potential profits, drug companies and the U.S. military forcibly vaccinated hundreds of thousands of soldiers and private contractors and failed to adequately monitor them for adverse side effects. Null concluded by offering "natural ways" for citizens to ward off ailments caused by bioweapons, including diet, detoxification, de-acidification, de-stressing, and herbal supplements like echinacea, garlic, vitamin A, and beta carotene.[44]

Just as Hooper's *The River* serves as the ultimate authority in the OPV AIDS hypothesis, Gary Matsumoto's 2004 *Vaccine A: The Covert Government Experiment That's Killing Our Soldiers and Why GI's Are Only the First Victims* offers a comprehensive analysis of the claimed link between anthrax vaccines and Gulf War Syndrome. Matsumoto was an NBC reporter who was embedded with the U.S. 10th Mountain Division and the 24th Mechanized Infantry Division before and during the Persian Gulf War. In the late 1990s, he became interested in the large numbers of veterans complaining about aching joints, rashes, fatigue, hair loss, sore gums, headaches, memory loss, and digestive problems. He spent six years pulling together the story of what he called "the secret activities of a few (not all) American military doctors, who, I came to realize, have been medically experimenting on troops for the past fifty years, almost without pause." Matsumoto claimed the sick veterans had been injected with vaccines that contained squalene, a natural organic compound sometimes used as an adjuvant in vaccines. Adjuvants are added to vaccines to help stimulate the body's immune system, thus increasing the vaccines' effectiveness by making the immune system respond more aggressively than it otherwise would. Drawing from research done at Tulane University, Matsumoto argued that the veterans were suffering from autoimmune disorders, which consisted of "damage that occurs when the immune system mistakenly identifies the body's own tissues as foreign matter and attacks it." He concluded that the lots of vaccines that contained squalene had initiated a series of autoimmune disorders, and he accused the United States federal government and the U.S. military of covering up the problem and continuing to use vaccines that contained squalene. Worse yet, he asserted that with funding from the National Institutes of Health, "scientists have formulated vaccines for flu, human papillomavirus (to prevent cervical cancer), malaria, HIV and herpes that also contain squalene." Why? According to Matsumoto, "There is some evidence that the corrupting influence of money has played a role in this."[45]

The allegation that vaccines caused Gulf War Syndrome brought together concerns from the political left and the political right. It included the by-then familiar claims that vaccines were injuring people because officials had not conducted the necessary safety studies and because profit-hungry pharmaceutical companies took shortcuts around safety procedures. The claims offered by advocates for the sick veterans are the height of American anti-vaccination sentiment, and they provide today's parents the assertions that they use to express their concerns about vaccines.

Two particularly relevant issues come to light around Gulf War Syndrome and the allegations that vaccines were either a cause of or a contributing factor in it. First, the emergence of the Gulf War Syndrome provides modern American anti-vaccinators the notion that vaccines—singularly, in combination with one another, or in combination with some other medicine or environmental factor—sometimes overwhelm children's' bodies and lead to a set of long-term health problems. Adjuvants and preservatives appear to be common culprits as authors have sought to identify the source of the problems.

Fears about the collective effects of vaccines and their components have coalesced into the common concern that systemic ailments may arise when immune systems are overwhelmed by vaccines, especially in the cases of young
children who receive multiple vaccines in a single visit to the doctor's office.
Autoimmune disorders—like lupus, multiple sclerosis, Guillain-Barré Syndrome, Crohn's disease, diabetes, and rheumatoid arthritis—and their symptoms are all discussed in alternative analyses of Gulf War Syndrome as well
as in concerns expressed by modern American anti-vaccinators. Vaccine-
induced autoimmune disorders—called vaccinosis—were first identified in
dogs and cats and discussed by Richard Pitcairn in *Prevention Magazine* in
1985. Pitcairn wrote, "The more I learn about the nature of the immune system, the more concerned I am about the increasing number of vaccine
viruses we are giving animals and possible repercussions that may result."
Vaccinosis and a general concern about vaccines soon became a central concern in the alternative veterinary community's notions about animal health.
The term *vaccinosis* appears to be working its way out of the alternative medical community and into the discussion about vaccine use in humans. Closely
related to this is the assertion that some people are genetically more vulnerable to the problems caused by exposure to certain agents.[46]

Second, there are strong allegations that financial motives played a substantial role in creating Gulf War Syndrome and continue to have an effect by
motivating authorities to ignore or dispute claims of a link between it and
vaccines. Null and many other authors have made pointed accusations that
retired Admiral William Crowe Jr., former head of the Joint Chiefs of Staff,
personally profited from his relationship with the U.S. military and his par-
tial ownership of the manufacturer of the anthrax vaccine. The Lansing,
Michigan-based company BioPort had a $45 million contract (which was
later increased by another $24.1 million) with the Pentagon to supply anthrax
vaccine. Null explains that Crowe "was given 12 percent to 13 percent of the
company in exchange for a 'token amount' and BioPort's use of his name." A
quick search of the words *william crowe bioport* on the Internet reveals thousands of hits on websites like 911review.org, whatreallyhappened.com, edu
cateyourself.org, and militarycorruption.com. As we will see, the claim that
financially motivated scientists and physicians are being allowed to shape
American vaccine policy to the detriment of our health (and to the benefits of
their wallets) is a central claim among modern American anti-vaccinators
and a concern frequently raised by vaccine-anxious parents.[47]

By the twenty-first century, vaccine-anxious parents had at their disposal a large collection of criticisms about vaccines, their manufacturers, American public health officials, and the federal government. We can identify a few general sources for these concerns, such as the longstanding criticism among members of the alternative health community and, at least in the case of Gulf War Syndrome, certain segments of the political right. For the critics who are energized against vaccines, the emergence of almost anything that resembles the broad range of ailments associated with vaccinosis is yet another problem caused by vaccines. As Abraham Maslow said in his 1966 book *The Psychology of Science*, "I suppose it is tempting, if the only tool you have is a hammer, to treat everything as if it were a nail." The anti-vaccinators who pound away at every issue that seems even tangentially linked to vaccines have amassed a very large collection of potential ills caused by the modern vaccine schedule.[48]

However passionate early critics of vaccines were, they had little influence on the average American throughout most of the twentieth century. But, by the mid-1990s their claims leaped into the mainstream by way of the mysterious origins of both HIV/AIDS and Gulf War Syndrome. By the late 1990s, modern concerns about vaccines were already in place: vaccines are not safe and they are not effective, we over-vaccinate, we have not done enough research on the long-term effects of vaccines, decisions are being made to advance some people's wealth rather than the public's health, and mainstream medicine ignores the many problems with the modern vaccine schedule. We need one more ingredient to understand the chaotic context and confusing set of claims that all American parents negotiate today in deciding whether and how to vaccine their children. Fringe anti-vaccination sentiment could only be fully imported into the mainstream with increasing concerns about autism.

3

Thimerosal and Autism

Today, U.S. parents worry that certain vaccines cause or trigger certain health problems. Of all these perceived adverse effects, none elicits more anxiety than the belief that vaccines might cause autism. Autism and the closely related diagnoses of Asperger's Syndrome and Pervasive Developmental Disorder—Not Otherwise Specified are collectively called Autism Spectrum Disorders or ASD. Informally, among members of the public and in the language of activist groups, they are simply grouped together under the label of autism.

The term *autism* was coined by Hans Asperger in 1938. Its modern use originated in a 1943 report by Leo Kanner of Johns Hopkins University Hospital about eleven children with remarkable similarities in their behaviors. Kanner described the children's disinterest in normal relationships with other people and their apparent desire for "aloneness" and "sameness." He concluded, "these children have come into the world with an innate inability to form the usual, biologically provided affective contact with people, just as other children come into the world with innate physical or intellectual handicaps." Throughout much of the twentieth century, reported cases of autism were incredibly rare, so much so that the American Psychiatric Association did not even include precise criteria for it in its *Diagnostic and Statistical Manual of Mental Disorders* until 1980. It took another decade before public schools in the United States began using the category of autism, which was followed by increasingly high rates of diagnoses. A broad range of impairments and capacities are associated with autism, from severe social impairment and mental disabilities to high functioning individuals with unusual interests or communication styles.[1]

As with other syndromes or disorders, autism is not considered a disease because medical science has not identified an underlying cause that explains the symptoms that usually occur together. Rather than being labeled as diseases, syndromes and disorders are constellations of symptoms that suggest the presence of an abnormality, an injury, or a disease. The symptoms that frequently occur in people diagnosed with autism include a lack of social skills and ability to interact easily with others, delayed development of speech, lack of imaginative play, a fixation on repetitive and ritualistic behaviors, and unusual eating habits. Today, parents usually identify symptoms of autism within the first three years of life. A formal diagnosis is based on a child's behavior rather than on an identified organic cause or a biological test. Over the last fifteen years there has been a substantial increase in the public's awareness of autism, and a number of therapies have emerged to treat children diagnosed with it. Researchers today believe what we call autism is caused by a complex set of interrelated genetic and environmental factors, making the search for a single cause or a single therapy futile.[2]

Concerns about autism are significantly heightened by a recent large increase in the number of children diagnosed with an Autism Spectrum Disorder. Some studies, such as one commissioned by the California legislature in 1999, reported that the number of children diagnosed as autistic nearly tripled from 1990 to 2000. In 2007, the CDC's Autism and Developmental Disabilities Monitoring Network reported that one in every one hundred fifty eight-year-old boys and girls in the United States had a diagnosable autism spectrum disorder. The CDC also reported that boys are four times more likely than girls to be diagnosed as autistic; one in ninety-four boys is diagnosed as autistic. In 2009, the CDC reported that the frequency of children diagnosed with an ASD in its most recent study was one in one hundred and ten, and as high as one in seventy boys. Shortly after the release of the movie *Rain Man* in 1988, a wave of public figures, including Dan Marino, Doug Flutie, and Don Imus, began discussing the "autism epidemic," and media outlets like the *New York Times*, CBS News, and *Time* were asking questions about the "shocking report" of a "mysterious upsurge" in autism and asserting that "cases of autism and closely related disorders like Asperger's are exploding in number, and no one has a good reason for it." Over the last several years, the assertion that new cases of autism have reached epidemic proportions has been accepted as a fact by a substantial number of Americans, and several recent books on the subject are based on an assumed epidemic of autism in the United States.[3]

Scientists now believe that genes exert significant influence in causing or making a child susceptible to autism. The first evidence for a genetic basis for autism came in a 1977 study that examined eleven pairs of identical twins and ten pairs of nonidentical twins in which at least one of the twins was diagnosed as autistic. The researchers found that in identical twins autism was diagnosed in both twins in over a third of the cases. Among the nonidentical twins, there was not a single case of both twins being diagnosed as autistic. More recent studies have supported the conclusion that there is a significant genetic component in the cause of autism, but precisely where in the genome the origins of autism reside is still unclear. The increasing tendency among health professionals to emphasize a genetic basis for autism problematizes the notion of an epidemic of autism; as pro-vaccine pundits have been quick to point out, it is impossible for a genetically based ailment to rapidly become epidemic.[4]

Environmental factors exerting influence from conception through early childhood have been widely suspected of being somehow involved in the emergence of autism, and the most recent studies suggest that they out-weigh genetic factors. Scientific investigations have raised concern about a number of potential causal influences in the environment, including second-hand smoke, poor ventilation in the home, vinyl chloride (which is used in PVC products like some flooring and furniture), nickel, pesticides, vitamin D deficiency, certain heavy metals like mercury and cadmium, rubella infection during pregnancy, air pollution, prenatal exposure to medications like thalidomide and valproic acid, and a number of different solvents used as degreasers or paint thinners. Some studies have concluded that environmental factors are most harmful when children are still in the womb, while others have examined early childhood exposure. Lately, a number of scientific papers suggest that autism is caused by a combination of genetic and environmental factors. In this model, some children are born genetically susceptible to some of the symptoms of autism and begin to show some of the symptoms that we associate with autism after being exposed to some sort of environmental influence.[5]

Over the last several years, dozens of articles in professional journals addressed the claim that there is some sort of epidemic of autism in the United States; most of them ardently disputed it. Scientists accept that there are people who have the symptoms associated with autism and are accurately diagnosed, and that there are probably other people who have some of the symptoms and are diagnosed with autism because of increased awareness and various social, parental, and institutional pressures. Most officials assert that these circumstances do not warrant the claim that there is an autism epidemic in the United States. Instead, a number of factors have combined to bring about the appearance of a rapid increase in the occurrence of autism when, in fact, autism is no more common today than it was in the past. Most significant among them is the fact that it was only recently that doctors had a clear set of criteria to use in diagnosing autism, and those criteria have substantially widened over the last several decades.

In 1980, the American Psychiatric Association's third edition of the *Diagnostic and Statistical Manual* (the *DSM-III*) required that a patient satisfy six mandatory criteria before being diagnosed on the autism spectrum, but the 1994 *DSM-IV* offered sixteen optional criteria of which only half had to be met. There was also a significant change in tone between the *DSM-III* and the *DSM-IV* that allowed clinicians to be much more inclusive in diagnosing autism. Moreover, there are emotional and sometimes even financial incentives that encourage parents to seek, and experts to diagnose, autism in a troubled or difficult child. Most authors have concluded, as Edward Campion did in his 2002 article in the *New England Journal of Medicine*, that the "increase is probably the result of better reporting and wider use of this diagnosis to describe children with unexplained cognitive and behavioral disorders." In short, in Campion's view, the wider definition of autism, the emergence of various incentives to diagnose a patient on the autism spectrum, the inaccurately low numbers of children who have autism in earlier studies, and the increasing public awareness of the symptoms associated with autism can easily lead one to assume, incorrectly, that there are far more children on the autism spectrum today than there were in the past.[6]

Occasionally we find scientists or medical experts who argue that there has been a rapid increase in the incidence, not just the diagnoses, of autism. Such claims are often offered by people with personal or professional links to individuals diagnosed with autism. This has been the basis for accusations of conflict of interest. Take, for example, an article in the *Journal of American Physicians and Surgeons* by F. Edward Yazbak, a retired pediatrician. Yazbak argues, "There has been a true and significant increase in autism" in the United States, and then asserts that "emerging evidence suggests some relationship between MMR and the thimerosal-containing vaccines and regressive autism." A "competing interests" statement reveals that "Dr. Yazbak is the grandfather of a boy with regressive autism, typical 'autistic' enterocolitis, and evidence of measles genomic RNA in the gutwall," all of which suggests that Yazbak accepts the claims that became popular in Britain in the late 1990s that the measles vaccine might cause gastrointestinal problems that could lead to developmental disorders. Critics assert that, because individuals like Yazbak have family members who are afflicted with autism, they cannot contribute to the scientific discussion about vaccines and autism. Following that logic, however, one would likewise be compelled to question claims made by any vaccine proponent whose child was not autistic.[7]

From a parent's point of view, I recognize what appear to be two distinct notions about autism. The first has emerged from the mainstream scientific and medical communities. It is characterized by descriptions of the complexity of autistic disorders, a general belief that both genetics and environmental factors are involved, and assertive statements that, as the Mayo Clinic's website authoritatively states, there is "no link between vaccines and autism." It recommends behavior, communication, and educational therapies as well as medications to control the severe behavioral problems sometimes associated with autism. It also states definitively, "There's no way to prevent autism."[8]

The second description of autism comes from proponents of alternative medicine—or, as its practitioners sometimes call it, the "biomedical approach"— and asserts that "the majority of children with autism are born healthy and neurologically normal but may have some genetic abnormalities that set them up for autism." It shares with mainstream medicine a belief in the complexity of autism spectrum disorders and agrees with its notion that both genetics and environmental factors play a role in the emergence of autism's symptoms in children. It differs considerably, though, in its range of acceptable treatments—of which alternative medicine offers many—as well as the methods for vetting treatments. As Robert W. Sears, a prominent advocate of the biomedical approach to autism, explained, "It focuses more on trial and error. . . . Because it almost always involves natural treatments, the error part of this trial-and-error approach is simply that the treatment doesn't work, not that it causes harm. The proof that something works is achieved more by consensus and not by the traditional scientific method." More significantly for our discussion, alternative health care providers roundly reject the mainstream medical community's belief that autism cannot be prevented. Instead, they assert, "biological, environmental, nutritional, allergic, and infectious factors contribute to autism," which means "prevention is possible by minimizing or eliminating as many of these biomedical factors as we can, from preconception through the first several years of life."[9]

Vaccines are an environmental influence that many alternative health care providers believe are a potential cause of or contributing factor to the symptoms associated with autism. None of the other potential causes of autism have captured the public's attention as powerfully as have the claims that routine childhood vaccines might be responsible for the apparent epidemic of autism in America, and about one-fifth of American parents believe that there is a causal link between vaccines and autism. The assertion that autism was somehow linked to vaccines emerged nearly simultaneously in the United States and in Britain from two very different sources and implicating two different causes. Their distinct origins and fundamentally different claims about exactly how vaccines might cause autism demonstrates just how anxious British and American parents had grown about vaccines and shows how easily they adopted an explanation that was critical of the modern vaccine schedule.

In the United States in the mid-1990s, public and professional concerns about thimerosal, a mercury-based preservative used in vaccines, prompted widespread discussion about its potentially harmful side effects. After decades of warnings from government agencies about the dangers of environmental toxins like mercury and lead, parents were shocked to learn that their physicians had been routinely injecting them and their children with vaccines that contained a mercury-based preservative. For parents, the rapid increase in the diagnoses of autism and concerns about thimerosal became linked.

The British vaccine/autism debate, which emerged in 1998, was originally unrelated to American concerns about thimerosal. It began when a research team at the Royal Free Hospital in London published an article in the *Lancet* suggesting a potential link between the measles, mumps, and rubella vaccine (MMR), gastrointestinal diseases, and developmental disorders like autism. Over the next decade, dozens of studies exploring the possibility of a link between the MMR vaccine and neurological disorders, including autism, concluded that there was no evidence whatsoever of a connection.

Since shortly after the turn of the twenty-first century, the mainstream American and British medical communities have agreed that there is no causal link between vaccines and the onset of symptoms of autism in otherwise healthy children. By 2009, the CDC could cite nine authoritative studies from researchers around the world concluding that there is no demonstrable link between vaccines and autism. Nevertheless, the public controversy continues. A 2008 survey of one thousand Americans found less than thirty-eight percent of them believe that there is no link between vaccines and autism. Britain's controversy over MMR and autism shared so many commonalities with Americans' concerns about thimerosal that shortly after the turn of the century, most Americans had effectively merged together the issues of the MMR vaccine, thimerosal, and autism. The ease with which these two controversies developed and merged tells us a great deal about the anxieties that many American and British parents feel about vaccines.[10]

Thimerosal and the Problem of Unintended Consequences

In 1997, in response to pressure from patient advocacy groups as well as researchers, physicians, and the pharmaceutical industry, Congress passed and President Clinton signed into law the U.S. Food and Drug Administration Modernization Act. According to the FDA's website, it was intended to enhance the "FDA's mission in ways that recognized the Agency would be operating in a 21st century characterized by increasing technology, trade and public health complexities." The massive reform required a number of changes to FDA policy; among them, it streamlined the drug approval process, increased patients' access to experimental drugs and medical devices, and abolished the longstanding law that prohibited pharmaceutical manufacturers from distributing information about the off-label uses for their drugs. It also ordered the creation of a list of drugs and foods that contained mercury compounds, requiring that the Secretary of Health and Human Services work with the FDA, the Institute of Medicine, and the National Academies of Sciences to conduct "a study of the effect on humans of the use of elemental, organic, or inorganic mercury when offered for sale as a drug or dietary supplement." One part of the study evaluated the use of mercury in drugs and supplements and the "adverse effects on health of children and other sensitive populations resulting from exposure to, or ingestion or inhalation of, mercury when so used." Finally, the act asked for opinions on the regulation of mercury that would "protect the health of children." The requirement that the FDA compile the list of mercury-containing foods and drugs came from an amendment attached to the bill by Frank Pallone, a Democratic congressman from a district in New Jersey that includes shore towns where mercury in fish was a significant environmental concern.[11]

It is hard to escape the irony of the unintended consequences of the FDA Modernization Act of 1997 on the public's anxieties about vaccines and autism. The act was passed as part of the National Partnership for Reinventing Government and was intended to make life-saving drugs more quickly available while simultaneously insuring and extending consumer protections and encouraging the development of new drugs. While it was never intended to stimulate parents' anxieties about vaccines, the act did just that. By speeding up the process for bringing new vaccines to market and by initiating an investigation into the potentially harmful effects of the various forms of mercury in food and drugs, the act alerted the public to the potential threat of the mercury that was—from their point of view—hidden in vaccines. At the same time, the number of new vaccines on the market drastically increased; recall the advertisement that appeared in *USA Today* when Annabelle was born, claiming that the CDC had tripled the number of vaccines children were to receive. The apparent rapid increase in diagnoses of autism, the underlying claims from anti-vaccinators, and the explosive increase in new vaccines that was created in part by the Modernization Act combined to create a wave of anxiety among American parents.[12]

Parents' concerns about the hidden risks to their children from mercury in vaccines came as the FDA and the Environmental Protection Agency campaigned to reduce pollution from environmental toxins like mercury, lead, and PCBs. Beginning in the mid-1950s, the United States passed a series of environmental acts, including the Air Pollution Control Act of 1955, the Clean Air Act of 1963, the Air Quality Act of 1967, the Clean Air Act Extension of 1970, and amendments to the Clean Air Act in 1997 and 1990. Throughout the second half of the twentieth century, Americans grew increasingly concerned about the potential health problems caused by environmental pollution, and public health campaigns aimed to educate parents about the long-term health effects of exposure to such dangerous toxins. Pregnant women were warned to avoid fish and shellfish that contain mercury because of the recognized harms it causes to babies' developing brains. Once born, children were still susceptible to damage from mercury from the environment, the foods they consumed, the medicines and vaccines they took, and even from breast milk.

In May of 1999, the FDA concluded its evaluation of mercury-containing foods and drugs and found that by six months of age infants could potentially receive as much as 187.5 micrograms of mercury from the vaccines against diphtheria, tetanus, pertussis, Hib, and hepatitis B. The Environmental Protection Agency (EPA) had set acceptable daily exposure levels of mercury at 0.1 microgram per day to each child's kilogram, which meant that the weekly mercury limit for a median-sized six-month-old girl was only 89 micrograms. The EPA's limits, however, are the lowest of any American or international agency, and have been estimated to have as much as a ten-fold safety factor. Nonetheless, researchers found that the thimerosal-containing vaccines significantly exceeded the EPA's calculated exposure limits for mercury.[13]

Parents came to understand that mercury was an ingredient in some childhood vaccines because of the use of thimerosal (sometimes spelled thiomersal), a preservative that has been used in many vaccines, medicines, and tattoo inks for over seven decades. After several episodes of bacterial contamination of vaccines caused illness and death in a small number of children in the United States and Australia in the 1930s, health officials and vaccine manufacturers began calling for the preservative to be used in all multiuse vaccine vials. Unlike most other preservatives of the time, thimerosal did not reduce the effectiveness of the vaccine, and it protected against fungal and viral growth in multiuse vials of vaccines, which are preferred by most physicians and health clinics because they are less expensive per dose and require less refrigerated storage space. By the end of the twentieth century, the preservative was used in almost three dozen different vaccines that were licensed and marketed in the United States. About half of the contents by weight of thimerosal is mercury. Given the FDA's recommended daily limits for mercury and the amount of mercury in various vaccines, it is possible for a median-sized six-month-old girl to be injected with twice the recommended limits of mercury in the course of receiving her routine childhood vaccines. It appears that in practice very few children actually get enough vaccines with mercury in them to reach or exceed the FDA's recommended limits over extended periods. However, for shorter periods, they probably do; a study published in the *Journal of Pediatrics* in 2000 of the infants who had received the hepatitis B vaccine within the first three days after birth—as Annabelle had—found that mean mercury blood levels increased substantially.[14]

In 1999, the FDA concluded its initial comprehensive review of the use of thimerosal in childhood vaccines by issuing a joint statement with the American Academy of Pediatrics (AAP) urging vaccine manufacturers to reduce or eliminate thimerosal from vaccines as quickly as possible. Even at that, officials stated that they found "no evidence of harm from the use of thimerosal as a vaccine preservative," and they were calling for its removal as a precautionary measure. Over the next several years, pharmaceutical companies developed, received approval for, and began selling thimerosal-free formulations of most of the major childhood vaccines. Today, the FDA reports, "all routinely recommended vaccines for American infants are available only as thimerosal-free formulations or contain only trace amounts of thimerosal, with the exception of inactivated influenza vaccine." By "available," the FDA means that thimerosal-free vaccines or vaccines with very low levels of thimerosal have been licensed and produced; that is no guarantee that a particular pediatrician will use them in the course of normal vaccinations. Even though most of the mercury has been removed from childhood vaccines, the issue continues to excite considerable public interest as well as a great deal of concern among parents.[15]

While parents and anti-vaccinationists typically talk about mercury as though all of its forms are essentially the same, each offering basically the same potential health risks, there are in fact three different types of mercury: elemental mercury, which is found in products like thermometers, florescent light bulbs, and amalgam dental fillings; organic mercury, which is used as a preservative and disinfectant in some vaccines and medicines; and nonelemental forms of inorganic mercury, which are used in batteries and some disinfectants. The mercury relevant to our discussion of vaccines is organic mercury, of which there are two principal types still in use: methylmercury and ethylmercury (a third type, phenylmercury, is a fungicide that has not been available since 1991). These compounds are composed of a mercury atom attached to a chain of carbon and hydrogen atoms—one carbon atom in methylmercury and two in ethylmercury. In thimerosal, the ethylmercury is incorporated in a larger organic molecule. Public health officials and vaccine advocates are quick to point out that most of the studies on mercury's health risks have examined methylmercury, while thimerosal contains ethylmercury.

Methylmercury is primarily created when burned fossil fuels, particularly coal, releases inorganic mercury into the atmosphere, which then finds its way into aquatic systems where organisms convert the inorganic mercury into methylmercury. It accumulates in the organisms and magnifies as it moves up the food chain, so that its highest concentrations are found in top-level aquatic predators, like tuna, walleye, largemouth bass, northern pike, swordfish, marlin, and shark. Once humans eat these organisms, the methylmercury is easily absorbed into the bloodstream and moves freely through the body, including across the blood-brain barrier and through the placenta, where developing fetuses absorb it. Scientific studies have shown that it causes cognitive and behavioral problems in humans, including reduced IQ, delayed development of language skills, lowered memory functions, and attention deficits. When authorities raise concerns about the health effects of mercury, they are talking specifically about methylmercury, and concerns about mercury's effects on human health as well as the bulk of their studies on the health effects of mercury are based on methylmercury.[16]

Unlike methylmercury, the ethylmercury in thimerosal appears to have little effect on our health and wellbeing because it is actively excreted by our digestive systems rather than accumulating the way methylmercury does. Although U.S. health authorities asked vaccine manufacturers to stop using thimerosal in childhood vaccines, researchers and physicians have been clear and assertive in their claims that thimerosal does not pose any risk to children. For example, in a 2006 statement on the subject, the World Health Organization stated that, on the basis of four independently conducted epidemiological studies in Britain, Northern Ireland, and Denmark, "the most recent pharmacokinetic and developmental studies do not support concerns over the safety of thiomersal (ethyl mercury) in vaccines. The committee concluded that there is no reason on the grounds of safety to change the current immunization practices with thiomersal-containing vaccines, as the risks are unproven." Likewise, the CDC explains, "Thimerosal does not stay in the body a long time so it does not build up and reach harmful levels. When thimerosal enters the body, it breaks down to ethylmercury and thiosalicylate, which are easily eliminated." Despite confidence that thimerosal presents no health risk whatsoever to the unborn, to children, or to adults, the CDC also reports, "in July 1999, the Public Health Service agencies, the American Academy of Pediatrics, and vaccine manufacturers agreed thimerosal should be reduced or eliminated in vaccines as a precautionary measure."

By 2004, a pile of scientific studies and associated papers demonstrated that researchers could find no causal relationship between any childhood vaccine or current vaccine component and the development of autism. The overwhelming consensus of the international medical and scientific communities is that in both the past and today, the presence of thimerosal in childhood vaccines presents no perceivable risk to our physical health or cognitive abilities, and numerous articles offer advice to physicians about how to best communicate this conclusion to parents.[17]

There are several reasons why parents have continued to be concerned about thimerosal despite the assured confidence expressed by the American and international public health community about the continued, albeit reduced, use of it in vaccines. First, the level of complexity, especially when one starts comparing the chemical formulations and potential health risks of ethylmercury to those of methylmercury, is so great that it is difficult for parents to develop any sense of confidence in the claims about health risks. For most parents, mercury is mercury, it is dangerous to their health and to the health, safety, and well being of their children, and it certainly should not be injected directly into their bodies in any form. This is understandable. After all, the EPA has set guidelines and carried out public education campaigns to convince people that mercury is a health risk—then, lo and behold, we learn that pediatricians are routinely injecting mercury into our children.

Second, the bold distinction that health officials draw between ethylmercury and methylmercury is perhaps not valid. At the very least, we can say that there is some evidence demonstrating that methylmercury is harmful, especially to young children, and some evidence that ethylmercury might not be as dangerous as methylmercury. In 2001, two years after the FDA, AAP, and the U.S. Public Health Service called on vaccine manufacturers to remove thimerosal from U.S.-licensed vaccines, the AAP's journal, *Pediatrics*, published "An Assessment of Thimerosal Use in Childhood Vaccines." The article's authors, three physicians working for the Food and Drug Administration, explained, "no controlled studies have been conducted to examine low-dose thimerosal toxicity in humans." However, they argued, in sharp contradiction to later claims by public health authorities and vaccine proponents, that "available data suggest that the toxicity of ethylmercury, the thimerosal metabolite, and methylmercury may be similar." This belief was based on research showing that "high-dose exposure to ethylmercury from thimerosal results in toxicity comparable to that observed after high-dose exposure to methylmercury," and involved recognition that the two compounds were chemically very similar. In the only animal study that compared the two forms of mercury, researchers concluded that the neurotoxicity of ethylmercury and methylmercury was similar. The authors concluded, "It appears reasonable to consider toxicity of the low doses of methylmercury and ethylmercury to be similar." A widely disseminated study analyzed the levels of mercury found in the blood and brains of infant monkeys exposed to methylmercury with those exposed to vaccines containing thimerosal. The authors found that, as public health officials and vaccine proponents had claimed, ethylmercury cleared from the monkey's systems about two and a half times faster than methylmercury. But, while they concluded that methylmercury was "not a suitable reference for risk assessment from exposure to thimerosal-derived ethylmercury," they were also critical of the Institute of Medicine's "decision to back away from the American Academy of Pediatrics goal" of removing thimerosal from all U.S.-licensed childhood vaccines. Later studies have come to the same conclusion—our bodies metabolize ethylmercury and methylmercury at different rates—but all have asserted the need for caution and additional research.[18]

Just how problematic is the fuzzy distinction between ethylmercury and methylmercury to parents who must make critical decisions about their children's vaccinations? Let us first recognize that ingestion or injection of mercury into our bodies in any form at any time carries risk of harm, even if it is a relatively small level of harm to our health or cognitive functions. High and very harmful amounts of methylmercury can build up in our bodies when we ingest contaminated food, which is unquestionably bad, especially for the neurological development of young children and for woman who are pregnant, could be pregnant, or are nursing. Then, let us accept that the ethylmercury in thimerosal is not as problematic for humans as is methylmercury because we are able to clear it from our systems in about week. Let us also accept that research shows that inoculating babies with thimerosal-containing vaccines does not "seem to raise blood concentrations of mercury above safe values in infants." Even accepting all of these assertions, as public health officials and vaccine proponents ask of us, we are left with a difficult question: Why are we injecting ethylmercury directly into our children's bodies in the critical early days and weeks and months of their lives? Even if the ethylmercury lingers in a baby's bloodstream and brain for a week or so (as some of the research demonstrates), why exactly are we pumping ethylmercury into infants? Parents are told, "Data from studies show no convincing evidence of harm caused by the low doses of thimerosal in vaccines." Yes, but how can it possibly be wise to directly inject mercury into infants' bodies? Over the last decade we have heard a chorus of reassuring claims from researchers, who say, "We could find no convincing evidence that early exposure to thimerosal had any deleterious effect on neurologic or psychological outcome." Vaccine manufacturers have continued to produce thimerosal-containing vaccines, most notably the annual flu vaccines, which are recommended for every child every year between six months and age six. The only reason pediatricians continue to purchase these vaccines, it would seem, is the convenience of saving refrigerator space in the clinic and the cost-savings that come from using multiuse vials of vaccines, which require antimicrobial agents to prevent the growth of bacteria. Instead of trying to argue away parents' concerns, why not just take all mercury out of all the vaccines?[19]

Another basis for parents' and activists' continuing concern about thimerosal in childhood vaccines is found in the contradictions so apparent in the words and actions of health authorities. On July 1, 1999, officials at the FDA sent letters to vaccine manufacturers asking them to stop using thimerosal in their U.S.-licensed vaccines. Officials stated that, based on their study of mercury compounds in drugs and food, they had "concluded that reducing or eliminating thimerosal from vaccines is merited," especially in vaccines administered to infants and children. Later that same month, the American Academy of Pediatrics and the U.S. Public Health Service issued a joint statement explaining that they and the vaccine manufacturers "agree that thimerosal-containing vaccines should be removed as soon as possible." They also recommended that, until mercury-free formulations of childhood vaccines were produced, "clinicians and parents can take advantage of the flexibility with the existing (vaccination) schedule to delay the hepatitis B" vaccination, which is normally given at birth. Three months later, the Centers for Disease Control and Prevention's Advisory Committee on Immunization Practices reaffirmed these recommendations.

In 1999, Neal Halsey, a pediatrician and current director of the Institute for Vaccine Safety at the Johns Hopkins Bloomberg School of Public Health, published an editorial in the *Journal of the American Medical Association* acknowledging, "The public has become intolerant of unnecessary exposure to real and theoretical risks for children from all sources, as evidenced by demands to make food products, toys, seat belts, and air bags as safe as possible." Therefore, he concluded, to "help maintain public confidence by demonstrating a commitment to provide the safest vaccines possible," authorities should insist on the complete removal of mercury from all vaccines just as they have sought to curtail industrial pollution of waterways with mercury. Clearly, at the turn of the twenty-first century, there was strong support for removing thimerosal from all U.S.-licensed childhood vaccines, and every major authority involved in the issue—the FDA, AAP, U.S. Public Health Service and the CDC—all supported its removal. Since then, thimerosal has been removed from most childhood vaccines, and it is true that there are now available thimerosal-free vaccines for all the mandated immunizations. But the influenza vaccine, which is recommended for children every year, still contains thimerosal, and there seems to be significant backsliding on pressure to remove thimerosal from all childhood vaccines.[20]

Instead of ardently standing by their calls that thimerosal be removed as a precautionary measure, authorities have shifted the bulk of their rhetoric to arguing that, despite common sense concerns about injecting children with mercury, there is no direct evidence that the thimerosal in childhood vaccines does any harm to children. For example, the AAP's website states, "Studies have found that there is no convincing scientific evidence that the low doses of thimerosal in vaccine causes harm." Likewise, the CDC's website asserts, "There is no convincing evidence of harm caused by the low doses of thimerosal in vaccines." Worse yet, health officials have demonstrated that they are willing to reintroduce thimerosal into the vaccines given to young children and pregnant women. For example, citing the need to quickly vaccinate everyone to avoid an influenza epidemic caused by H1N1 in 2009, health officials in Washington suspended their self-imposed rule preventing the administration of thimerosal-containing vaccines to pregnant women and children under age of three. A *Seattle Times* story received over 100 comments online, most of them critical of the Washington Health Department's decision including one that began, "You're freakin' kidding me!!" Another said, "Isn't it a bit odd that our government says pregnant women should avoid eating too much fish because the mercury levels are too high??? And then they recommend getting shot up with a mercury containing vaccine." From a parent's point of view, it seems that health authorities have replaced the principle of prudence with the mantra of "thimerosal in vaccines is (probably) safe." Why not just get rid of thimerosal instead of fighting an uphill battle over the supposed differences between ethylmercury and methylmercury and claims that low amounts of thimerosal have not shown to pose demonstrable risks to children's health and well-being?[21]

Finally, many parents and anti-vaccination authors continue to be concerned about thimerosal in childhood vaccines because the symptoms of mercury poisoning look so much like autism. They include angry fits, memory loss, sleep disturbance, loss of self-control, difficulty in learning, and a tendency toward repetitive behaviors, intestinal problems, and headaches.

Anti-vaccination authors have made much of the similarities between autism and mercury poisoning. These similarities were, in fact, the basis for what the CDC called the "precautionary measure" of asking manufacturers to remove thimerosal from vaccines in 1999. Add to this that parents have a relativistic notion of their child's health. When they are told that their child has received a vaccine that contained mercury, they are compelled to ask themselves, how much smarter, happier, well behaved, or better adjusted could my child have been had he or she not been injected with vaccines that contain mercury?[22]

The collective response of the American health care community to concerns about thimerosal in childhood vaccines both past and present has been, at best, dismissive. Their responses have relied on citations of epidemiological studies and case analyses that have all concluded there is no evidence that mercury-containing vaccines cause neurological problems in children. They have stressed that the known risks from vaccine-preventable communicable diseases far outweigh even the theoretical risks of the mercury-based preservatives that are used in vaccines. They frame the argument as if the thimerosal itself was a necessary ingredient and the choice was between vaccinating with thimerosal-containing vaccines or not vaccinating at all. In fact, aside from economic concerns, there is no solid reason why American children should not each be vaccinated with single-use vials, which would entirely eliminate the need for thimerosal in childhood vaccines.[23]

Despite these ardent claims—perhaps to some degree because of them—parents' common-sense concerns about injecting their children with vaccines that contain mercury continue, and the public controversy rages on. By virtue of their unwillingness to engage with parents' concerns and, for the moment, see past their rigid, normative notions of public health, physicians and public health officials have effectively handed the debate over to polemicists and thrown vaccine-anxious parents into the arms of anti-vaccinators.

Origins of the Public Controversy over Thimerosal

In the late 1990s, when increasing numbers of American parents first grew concerned about the mercury used in some routine childhood vaccines, they had at their disposal a set of arguments, ready-made by the alternative medicine community and honed to a sharp edge by the controversies over the origins of HIV/AIDS and Gulf War Syndrome. Vaccines, according to their critics, were unsafe, untested, and ineffective. The parents who imagined the

dangerous mercury floating in those little multiuse vials found these arguments incredibly alluring. Given health officials' sometimes contradictory
and often confusing stance on thimerosal at the turn of the century as well as
their dictatorial attitudes about the absolute necessity of universal vaccination, the claims and personal support offered by the anti-vaccinators in the
alternative medicine community welcomingly embraced anxious parents. To
solidify the opinions of multitudes of middle class parents against the one-
size-fits-all vaccination schedule, what was needed was a series of newsworthy
events and a handful of mainstream leaders to thrust anti-vaccination rhetoric
and concerns about autism into the limelight. These necessary ingredients
first emerged at the start of the twenty-first century with Dan Burton.

Congressman Dan Burton, the Republican representative from the Fifth
Congressional District of Indiana, has been a member of Congress since the
early 1980s. Born in Indianapolis and raised in a family torn by domestic vio-
lence, Burton worked as a golf caddy to make ends meet, then attended Indiana University for a year and the Cincinnati Bible Seminary for another
before becoming a real estate broker and insurance agent. On and off from
the late 1960s through the early 1980s he served in the Indiana House of Representatives. In 1983, he was elected to the U.S. House of Representatives, where
he has been a consistent supporter of the conservative agenda. He has a 100
percent prolife voting record, and he has received the highest possible rating
from the Gun Owners of America.

Burton has long been a supporter of causes associated with alternative
medicine and a critic of mainstream medicine. In the 1970s, when he was an
Indiana state senator, he participated in a campaign that was strongly endorsed by the John Birch Society (a right-wing political advocacy group that
calls for limited government) to legalize the sale of laetrile, a sham cancer
therapy that was made from apricot pits. In the 1990s, his wife was diagnosed
with breast cancer. She sought treatment from Georg Springer, an immunol-
ogist whose research on cancer treatments has been heralded by members of
the alternative medicine community. The FDA blocked Springer's cancer
vaccine trial from proceeding, a move that angered Burton and may help explain his tendency to attack the FDA and the mainstream scientific and medical communities. As a populist and a supporter of restricted government
influence, Burton "felt that the government had no place telling people what
cures to seek."[24]

Burton's animosity against government regulatory agencies and his apparent appreciation for alternative medicine was pushed further when two of his grandchildren experienced health and developmental complications after receiving routine vaccinations. In 1993, as Burton's daughter, Danielle Burton-Sarkine, tells it, her five-week-old daughter began screaming and crying inconsolably shortly after receiving a dose of hepatitis B vaccine. After hours of crying, the baby stopped breathing. Danielle started CPR, and the baby began breathing again just as the paramedics arrived. The baby spent three and a half weeks in the hospital recuperating before being sent home apparently free of any lingering health problems. In 1998, Burton's two-year old grandson, Christian, was vaccinated against diphtheria, pertussis, tetanus, measles, mumps, rubella, hepatitis B, *Haemophilus influenzae* type B, and polio in a single office visit to his pediatrician. Soon after, according to Congressman Burton and his daughter, Christian was diagnosed with mild to moderate autism.[25]

In 2000, a year after American health authorities made their public pronouncements asking vaccine manufacturers to remove thimerosal from childhood vaccines, Burton exercised his authority as chairman of the Committee on Government Reform to open a series of hearings on vaccines, mercury, and autism. Over the next three years, Burton used the hearings as a platform both to publicize the alleged links between autism and mercury in vaccines and to grill officials from the public health community. In his opening statement to one of the hearings, he said, "My only grandson became autistic right before my eyes—shortly after receiving his federally recommended and state-mandated vaccines. Without a full explanation of what was in the shots being given, my talkative, playful, outgoing healthy grandson Christian was subjected to very high levels of mercury through his vaccines. He also received the MMR vaccine. Within a few days he was showing signs of autism."[26]

Burton's congressional hearings were carefully planned and included many parents of children with autism. One reporter described them as "just plain folks whose honesty seemed unimpeachable." After the hearing began, hundreds of parents contacted Burton asking to give testimony, and Burton included many of them. His opening statement at the hearings that took place in April of 2000 described them one after another, beginning with another description of Burton's grandson, Christian, who was born healthy, but "then, his mother took him for his routine immunizations and all of that changed." Shelly Reynolds from the activist organization Unlocking Autism, had displayed "thousands of pictures of autistic children" at a rally earlier that week and told the committee how "forty-seven percent of the parents who provided these pictures felt that their child's autism was linked to immunizations." Liz Burt described how her five-year-old son was developing normally until, at "15 months, following his MMR vaccine, he began to regress." Burton invited Kenneth Curtis, a local radio personality, to talk about being the parent of an autistic child, as well as one of his constituents, James Smythe of Carmel, Indiana, to "share how, through properly looking at autism as an illness, and addressing that illness, his son is improving." He invited William Danker, whose thirteen-year-old daughter had autism, to talk about "the battles of getting adequate education through the public school system." Burton also brought in Andrew Wakefield and John O'Leary, whom we will meet in the next chapter, to testify about the potential dangers of the combined MMR vaccine and their efforts to treat children with neurological problems they believed are caused by endemic measles infections in their intestinal systems.[27]

In addition to providing a venue for a public recognition of the difficulties autism presented to parents and the children diagnosed with it, the hearings gave Burton the opportunity to interrogate the health authorities of whom he was so critical. Burton's anger toward them was obvious when he announced at a June 2002 hearing, "I'm so ticked off about my grandson, and to think that the public-health people have been circling the wagons to cover up the facts! Why it just makes me want to vomit!" Throughout the hearings he aggressively questioned government scientists, he accused many of them of bad faith and of conflicts of interest, and he sometimes even threatened to cut their funding if they did not provide him with the research results he wanted. At one meeting, he slammed to the desk a recently released report from the Institute of Medicine that concluded there was no link between the MMR vaccine and autism and, according to an account of the scene in the *Journal of the American Medical Association*, he "shouted, red-faced, 'You don't know there's no link, do you? Do you?'" Repeatedly, the committee urged the removal of thimerosal from all vaccines and called for additional research on autism. It lambasted federal agencies for their inattentiveness to the problem. Burton's 2003 "Mercury in Medicine" report to the U.S. House of Representatives criticized the FDA for acting "too slowly to remove ethylmercury from over-the-counter products." It called the Department of Health and Human Service's efforts to remove thimerosal from vaccines "not sufficiently aggressive," and charged that the CDC's "failure to state a preference for thimerosal-free vaccines in 2000 and again in 2001 was an abdication of their responsibility." In a clear demonstration of how earlier concerns about Gulf War Syndrome impacted the modern American anti-vaccination movement, Burton recommended that, among other things, "Congress should direct the National Institutes of Health to give priority to research projects studying causal relationships between exposure to mercury, methylmercury, and ethylmercury to autism spectrum disorders, attention deficit disorders, Gulf War Syndrome, and Alzheimer's Disease."[28]

After the media exposure about the challenges faced by parents of children with autism and the alleged link between vaccines and autism, the next most significant product of Burton's hearings was his exposure of the potential conflicts of interest that exist in the formulation of American vaccine policy, the research and manufacture of vaccines, and the incredible profits available for pharmaceutical companies and their employees. For example, the committee's report from 2000 reviewed the history of the vaccine RotaShield (the rotavirus vaccine that appeared to cause a very small increase in the number of intussusception cases). It found that the "conflict of interest rules employed by the FDA and the CDC have been weak, enforcement has been lax, and committee members with substantial ties to pharmaceutical companies have been given waivers to participate in committee proceedings."[29]

Burton has made it difficult for many people to accept him as a hero because he has been the target of a number of critical allegations of misconduct and conflict of interest. At the time of his investigation into links between vaccines and autism, Burton's daughter had filed an autism claim with the U.S. Office of Special Masters, the so-called vaccine court in which Americans who have been injured by vaccines can seek financial compensation. Burton never disclosed this fact during the hearings, and critics have asserted that Burton's hearings provided testimony useful in his daughter's suit and legitimacy for her claims. In 1998, a *New York Times* editorial called on Burton to resign as chairman of House Government Reform and Oversight Committee for being "an impediment to a serious investigation of the 1996 campaign finance scandals." To complicate matters further, Burton's "legislative jihad against vaccines," as one commentator called it, began shortly after Burton admitted to fathering a child in an extramarital affair in the early 1980s and to paying child support. Burton had been an active participant in the impeachment of President Clinton, was very critical of the president's re-lationship with Monica Lewinsky, and told the editorial board of the *India-napolis Star* that he thought the president was a "scumbag." So, news of Bur-ton's extramarital affair sparked widespread accusations of hypocrisy.[30]

In 2009, as officials worried about the spread of H1N1, several other prom-inent members of the American political right publicized their refusal to be vaccinated against it. In the midst of debates over national health care and accusations of the rationing of health care and "death panels," Rush Lim-baugh made headlines by announcing that he would not get the H1N1 influ-enza vaccine. "Screw you, Ms. Sebelius," he said, referring to Secretary of Health and Human Services, Kathleen Sebelius. "You'll be healthier," he told his audience, if you don't listen to the government. "All I see is a bunch of typical government panic and hype." Fox News personality Glenn Beck made similar assertions when he told viewers he wanted the "U.S. out of my blood-stream." The libertarian, nonpartisan Bill Maher told followers that people who get the flu shots are "idiots." On the his HBO show Bill Maher had a heated discussion with Republican Senator (and physician) Bill Frist about the H1N1 vaccine in which he downplayed the threat the flu presented to the general population and said, "I would never get a swine flu vaccine or any vaccine. I don't trust the government, especially with my health."[31]

The political and social movement against vaccines has not been the pur-view solely of members of the political right. Its bipartisan appeal has in-creased its potency as a force in modern American politics. Members of the political right like Burton attacked federal health authorities with their con-cerns about vaccines on the same grounds and with the same vigor they use to support other aspects of the conservative political agenda, including limit-ing government and extending personal liberties. At the same time, members of the political left have been animated by concerns about what is "natural" and about the abuses of industry and large corporations. Left-leaning Ameri-cans also often align their concerns about the contents of vaccines with advo-cacy for environmental causes. Nowhere do you see this more clearly presented than in the work of Robert F. Kennedy Jr.

Kennedy is an attorney and cohost of a weekly radio program on the lib-eral talk radio network Air America. He has devoted the last quarter-century of his career to environmental issues, especially to protection of water qual-ity. His concerns about mercury pollution from power plants led him to be-come interested in the alleged connection between the mercury used in thimerosal in vaccines and neurological problems in American children. The issue linked his environmental concerns with his penchant for attacking industry in the name of consumer safety and environmental protection. In June 2005 he published "Deadly Immunity" in *Rolling Stone* and alleged a government cover-up of the link between mercury and autism. According to Kennedy, in June 2000, a group of top government scientists and health officials gathered for a meeting at the remote Simpsonwood conference center in Norcross, Georgia. The CDC had convened a meeting of fifty-two invitation-only attendees, and "all of the scientific data under discussion, CDC officials repeatedly reminded the participants, was strictly 'embargoed.' There would be no making photocopies of documents, no taking papers with them when they left." They had met to hear and discuss the findings of Thomas Verstraeten, a CDC epidemiologist who had analyzed the medical records of one hundred thousand children and concluded that thimerosal "appeared to be responsible for a dramatic increase in autism and a host of other neurological disorders." The participants were alarmed and, according to Kennedy "spent most of the next two days discussing how to cover up the damaging data." When Verstraeten finally published his findings, Kennedy claimed, "he had gone to work for GlaxoSmithKline and reworked his data to bury the link between thimerosal and autism." The Simpsonwood meeting, as it has come to be called, is believed by many vaccine critics to be among the many examples of government complicity in the poisoning of children with thimerosal.[32]

Kennedy claims there is a generation of Americans—those born between 1989 and 2003—who "received heavy doses of mercury from vaccines." The increasing number of vaccines introduced in the late 1980s and early 1990s combined with the increasing use of thimerosal in vaccines led to what one school nurse had described to Burton's House Government Reform Committee in 1999 as a massive number of children with neurological problems overwhelming teachers and administrators in the elementary grades. Kennedy quoted her remarks from the congressional testimony: "Vaccines are supposed to be making us healthier; however, in twenty-five years of nursing I have never seen so many damaged, sick kids. Something very, very wrong is happening to our children." Kennedy attacked claims that there were not in fact more children with autism, rather only more children being diagnosed with autism. He quoted Boyd Haley, a professor of chemistry at the University of Kentucky, who told Burton's committee, "If the epidemic is truly an artifact of poor diagnosis, then where are all the twenty-year-old autistics?"

Kennedy blamed the problem on industry's profit motives and the much higher number of vaccines the average American child now receives. Thimerosal allows pharmaceutical companies to package vaccines in multiple use vials, which he said "cost half as much to produce as smaller, single-dose vials."

Kennedy relied heavily on the work done by Mark Geier and his son David Geier, both of whom have been active vaccine critics and have testified on behalf of plaintiffs in nearly a hundred vaccine injury cases. The Geiers have been targets of aggressive criticism from the AAP, a judge from the vaccine court, and other scientific authorities. For example, when the Institute of Medicine released its 2004 vaccine safety report, it described two studies by the Geiers and dismissed them both, describing one as "characterized by serious methodological flaws" and saying that their analytic methods were nontransparent and their results uninterpretable, and "therefore non-contributory with respect to causality." Like Kennedy, the Geiers believe the scientific evidence suggesting that thimerosal causes autism is conclusive, and they have published several papers arguing that thimerosal is in fact the cause of neurodevelopmental disorders. In an interview with the *New York Times* in 2005, Mark Geier said that public health officials are "just trying to cover it up." Kennedy's accusations and his apparent alignment with anti-vaccine authors were met by counterattacks suggesting that he had made a number of gross factual errors. The current online version of the *Rolling Stone* story includes a long list of clarifications and corrections.[33]

A month after his *Rolling Stone* article appeared, Kennedy was a guest on the Jon Stewart talk show. During his seven-minute segment, he asserted his claims that thimerosal had created a generation of neurologically damaged children and that both the federal regulators and the pharmaceutical industry were involved in a massive cover-up. He explained that between 1989 and 2003,

Almost all of our vaccinations included a material called thimerosal. . . . We saw during that period a dramatic increase in neurological disorders among American children. Today, one in every six children born during that period has some sort of neurological disorder—speech delay, language delay, dyslexia and at the opposite end of the range, autism. In 1988, before they started adding all these vaccines, one in every 2,500 children had autism. Today, one in 166 have autism and there is very, very strong science, really overwhelming science, linking those autism rates to the thimerosal that was in the vaccines.

The thimerosal, people should know, has been removed from most of the vaccines in America. We still have it in the flu vaccine and one or two others.

Kennedy's strong assertions about a link between autism and thimerosal led
Stewart to ask, "Why is there a fight?" Kennedy explained that the refusal by
federal regulators and the pharmaceutical companies to accept the apparently obvious link between autism and thimerosal was based on concerns
about litigation: "This is literally trillions of dollars in damages." There is
also, he said, "a concern with the scientists at CDC and the FDA . . . who
green-lighted the autism. . . . How many of us would want to admit that a
decision was made that poisoned a whole generation of American children?"
Finally, federal agencies and drug companies "want to make sure that people
don't get scared off from vaccines." But, he concluded with a veiled reference
to his claims about the Simpsonwood conference, "people are going to be
frightened of vaccines if they don't trust the federal regulators to be honest
with the American people. The biggest threat to our vaccine program is that
these people have now been caught red-handed conspiring to hide this information from the American people."[34]

Kennedy's assertions and accusations added an unusual twist to a heated
political dispute over science in which the political left attacked the right as
being antiscience. In the run-up to the 2004 presidential elections, critics of
the Bush administration had launched a number of claims that it had inappropriately "politicized science" by manipulating funding and research results in ways that privileged their policies. The Bush administration had been
attacked for installing former lobbyists and industry spokespeople in high-
ranking federal positions. In 2004, the Union of Concerned Scientists issued
a scathing report charging that the administration "has suppressed or dis-
torted the scientific analyses of federal agencies to bring these results in line
with administration policy," and that "irregularities in the appointment of
scientific advisors and advisory panels are threatening to upset the legally
mandated balance of these bodies." For the most part, claims that the Bush
administration had inappropriately politicized science focused on environmental issues, abstinence-only education, and stem cell research. Kennedy's
attacks, however, split the left/right divide by asserting that the anti-vaccinators
were on the side of good science and that health officials were blindly
and dogmatically ignoring the overwhelming scientific evidence of a link
between thimerosal and autism. "If you actually read the science," he told Jon

Stewart, "the science is overwhelming that there is a link between autism and the thimerosal." At the end the decade, vaccine proponents had begun efforts to turn the claims of politicization in their favor by asserting that anti-vaccinators were promoting fallacies in order to advance their claims about the supposed dangers of vaccines. For example, a November 2009 article in *Wired* that attacked anti-vaccinators' claims as unscientific generated more mail—most of it positive—than any other story ever published by the magazine.[35]

By the end of 2005, the American controversy over vaccines, thimerosal, and autism had grown so heated that health officials began expressing concerns about their own safety. The CDC reported it had received "a barrage of threatening letters and phone calls" which led them to increase security around their offices and to instruct employees on safety issues, "including how to respond if pies are thrown in their faces." One vaccine expert emailed colleagues saying that she "felt safer working at a malaria field station in Kenya than she did at the agency's offices in Atlanta." At a 2006 meeting of the Advisory Committee on Immunization Practices—the CDC committee principally responsible for setting the American vaccine schedule—a hundred protestors shouted accusations and slurs at some of the committee members. The scientists and physicians who evaluated claims about thimerosal and autism reported receiving threatening emails and phone calls. Paul Offit, a pediatrician, professor of vaccinology at the University of Pennsylvania, chief of the Division of Infectious Diseases, and director of the Vaccine Education Center at the Children's Hospital of Philadelphia—and one of the most ardent proponents of the modern vaccine schedule—began his recent book, *Autism's False Prophets*, by admitting, "I get a lot of hate mail. Every week people send letters and emails calling me 'stupid,' 'callous,' an 'SOB,' or 'a prostitute.'" Offit went on for several pages describing the threats he received, including veiled threats to his family.[36]

By the start of 2006, the American controversy over thimerosal in vaccines seemed to have reached a stalemate that persists today. Regulatory officials nearly universally assert that authoritative studies have failed to show any link between thimerosal and neurological disorders like autism. Nonetheless, they say, as a precautionary measure they have called for the production of thimerosal-free vaccines, which reduce the amount of the preservative in childhood vaccines by about ninety-eight percent. Many parents, however, are unconvinced by health officials' claims about both the past and present safety of vaccines. Large numbers of parents believe their children's current developmental or neurological problems are the result of vaccines or their components, and many more express serious reservations about the current vaccine regime despite the consistent assurances of American health officials. As Melinda Wharton, the deputy director of the National Immunization Program told a gathering of immigration officials in 2005, "It's an era where it appears that science isn't enough."[37]

Wharton was right.

4

MMR and Autism

The British vaccine controversy focused on the combined vaccine against measles, mumps, and rubella and the allegation that it causes, triggers, or exacerbates symptoms associated with autism. As with thimerosal and autism in the United States, health officials in Britain quickly produced evidence that there was no causal link between the vaccine and autism, and they rigorously disputed any claim of a connection. For vaccine-anxious parents who found vindication in the claim that the vaccine against measles, mumps and rubella might cause autism, however, no amount of scientific refutation of the work was persuasive.

In Britain, parents' anxieties about vaccines were piqued after Andrew Wakefield, a British academic gastroenterologist, suggested that the measles, mumps and rubella vaccine (MMR) be split into three separate vaccines because the combined vaccine might cause gastrointestinal difficulties that could lead to neurological problems like autism. In 1987, Wakefield arrived at the Royal Free Hospital in London to head the Inflammatory Bowel Disease (IBD) Study Group. From the late 1980s through the mid-1990s, he received significant funding from pharmaceutical companies and charities in support of his work, which focused on identifying the causes of inflammatory bowel diseases. Wakefield and his colleagues in the Inflammatory Bowel Disease Study Group published research that suggested that ailments like ulcerative colitis and Crohn's disease might be caused by a virus or multiple viruses, possibly in concert with a genetic predisposition or with other environmental factors. By the early 1990s, the IBD researchers had narrowed their search to one specific virus and one particular form of IBD; their research had led them to believe that the measles virus was responsible for triggering, causing, or helping to cause Crohn's disease. Between 1993 and 1997 they adapted their hypothesis to include the claim that not just the measles virus, but perhaps also the measles vaccine, could play a role in the onset of Crohn's disease. In February 1998 Wakefield, in collaboration with a dozen other colleagues, published a paper in the *Lancet*, Britain's premier medical journal, which linked chronic intestinal disorders with autism and asserted that symptoms for both began shortly after patients received the combined measles-mumps-rubella vaccine. With this publication, the public controversy in Britain over an alleged link between the MMR vaccine and autism began.[1]

Wakefield would later coin the term *autistic enterocolitis* to describe the form of IBD he believed was in some way caused by the MMR vaccine, which he believed in turn caused neurological problems that are consistent with autism. The controversy developed slowly, and we are able to follow it step-by-step, article-by-article, throughout the early and mid-1990s. By the end of the decade, the relatively small group of researchers engaged in the discussion grew into small armies of polemicists from various clinical and academic specialties, all of them publishing voluminously on the topic.

By 2002, the scientific and medical communities in Britain and the United States concluded that Wakefield's hypothesis was incorrect—in fact, there was no causal association between the MMR vaccine and autism. Soon after, Wakefield left Britain surrounded by considerable public controversy—made worse by charges of professional misconduct—and immigrated to the United States. In America, he found significantly more public support for his claims about a link between vaccines and autism, and he has continued both his private practice and his public advocacy for autistic children and their parents. In the United States as in Britain, the weight of opinion within the medical and scientific communities has remained steadfastly opposed to Wakefield's claims about the potential of vaccines, in particular the MMR vaccine, to cause autism.

Despite the central role that he has taken in the modern vaccine debates—and unlike the some of the chiropractors we met in an earlier chapter—Wakefield is not an opponent of vaccines. To the contrary, he has repeatedly stated his belief that vaccines are an important tool in preserving an individual's health and in protecting the nation's public health. As with Robert F. Kennedy Jr.'s criticisms of officials' attitude toward thimerosal, Wakefield argues that if we want to maintain high levels of vaccine compliance, we need to be especially careful about maintaining the public's confidence in their safety. From our perspective, Wakefield is significant not because his claims about autistic enterocolitis are correct, but because of the passion that his work has aroused, both for and against his claims. The evolution of Wakefield's thinking about the potential link between the MMR vaccine and developmental disorders reveals the complexity of the scientific claims as well as the many competing political and professional interests in modern vaccine controversies. It also demonstrates how these complex issues were boiled down to the simple claim that the MMR vaccine caused autism.

Wakefield's Hypothesis

In the late 1980s, Wakefield and his colleagues at the Royal Free Hospital first came to believe certain that inflammatory bowel diseases were linked to one or more viruses that seemed common in the bodies and diseased cells of patients with the ailment. In papers that appeared in the *Lancet*, the *Journal of Gastroenterology*, and the *Journal of Medical Virology*, they described how they had used microscopic techniques to analyze samples of intestinal tissue from patients who had been diagnosed with the two most common forms of IBD, Crohn's disease and ulcerative colitis. In their first paper on the subject, they concluded that the disease was in some way related to or caused by a series of multifocal gastrointestinal infarctions—small areas of the intestine that died because they lacked adequate blood supply. Another paper, published in 1990, suggested that the majority of the granulomas, nodules that form when the immune system attempts to fight off something that has activated it, originate within the blood vessels of the intestines. They had not, however, identified the root cause of the diseased sections of the intestine that led to Crohn's disease or ulcerative colitis.[2]

In the early 1990s, the Wakefield group switched from using microscopic techniques to examine diseased cells from the intestinal track to a relatively new laboratory technique, polymerase chain reaction (PCR). Invented in the early 1980s, PCR is a laboratory method for creating large numbers of exact copies of a section of a strand of DNA by directing the DNA to undergo repeated cycles of duplication. Kary Mullis, the technique's originator, described it this way: "Beginning with a single molecule of the genetic material DNA, the PCR can generate one hundred billion similar molecules in an afternoon. The reaction is easy to execute. It requires no more than a test tube, a few simple reagents, and a source of heat." PCR's value for Wakefield's research team rested on its ability to serve as a virus detector of sorts. Viruses consist of genetic material in the form of either DNA or RNA surrounded by a protective coat of proteins. If ailments like ulcerative colitis or Crohn's disease originated with a virus or with the interaction of multiple viruses in a patient's body, the researchers should be able to detect trace amounts of the virus in the diseased cells. By subjecting laboratory samples from patients with various forms of IBD to PCR and comparing them to similar samples from healthy patients, researchers could search for certain virus DNA and possibly uncover clues about potential causes of the diseases.[3]

The Wakefield group had reason to suspect there might be a link between viruses and intestinal diseases. Specifically, they were interested in an order of viruses called Herpesvirus, which includes herpes simplex virus 1 (which causes cold sores), herpes simplex virus 2 (which causes genital herpes), the varicella zoster virus (better known as the virus that causes chickenpox and shingles), the Epstein Barr virus (which causes mononucleosis), and cytomegalovirus (which causes a mononucleosis-like ailment). Other scientists had shown that some members of the Herpesvirus order were linked to ulcerative colitis. People with active ulcerative colitis, in fact, had elevated levels of antibodies for certain Herpesviruses. Likewise, people with severe ulcerative colitis have been found to have Herpesvirus inclusion bodies, the components that make up the protein shells of Herpesviruses and indicate a site where the virus is multiplying. Laboratory experiments had shown that Herpesviruses infect the thin layer of cells lining the interior of blood vessels and can cause functional changes in the cells similar to the changes seen in patients with ulcerative colitis. Herpesviruses can also produce the proteins cells use to signal one another to become inflamed and encourage white blood cells to adhere to an area. Both inflammation and accumulation of white blood cells are found in patients with active ulcerative colitis, all of which suggests a possible role for Herpesviruses in the development of ulcerative colitis.[4]

Motivated by this research, in the early 1990s Wakefield's IBD group began using PCR to detect the presence of DNA from the Herpesvirus in tissues taken from people with ulcerative colitis and Crohn's disease. Specifically, they looked for the presence of cytomegalovirus, varicella zoster virus, and Epstein Barr virus; they found that nearly fifty percent of the people with ulcerative colitis also tested positive for all three viruses. In contrast, only fourteen percent of the people with Crohn's disease and five percent of the healthy control subjects tested positive for all three. They concluded that "the high prevalence of DNA from multiple Herpesviruses in ulcerative colitis suggests a possible synergistic role for these viruses in the pathogenesis of the disease either in a primary or in a secondary role." Nonetheless, not all people who harbored the viruses contracted ulcerative colitis, so the group posited that perhaps "a genetic susceptibility predisposes certain individuals to develop the disease following exposure to a commonly occurring stimulus." This initial research conducted by Wakefield and his group generated no controversy whatsoever. It fit well with earlier research on the possible involvement of viruses in Crohn's disease. Nonetheless, the group's suggestion that some combination of the viruses and a genetic susceptibility were correlated with ulcerative colitis laid the foundation for Wakefield's later concerns about the MMR vaccine, as the group's line of inquiry exposed them to earlier research that had produced case reports of autistic-like syndromes in children affected with some of the Herpesviruses they were studying. The Herpesviruses were just one of several that the team considered in their efforts to find the cause of inflammatory bowel diseases. Measles, and eventually the measles vaccine, was another.[5]

Wakefield and six of his colleagues published the first claims about a relationship between measles and IBD in 1993. The research team examined tissues from people with Crohn's diseases and compared them with tissues from healthy subjects using two methods, in situ hybridization and immunohistochemistry, both of which allowed them to determine whether or not genetic material from the measles virus was present in the samples. Because measles is an RNA virus, the PCR techniques the team employed to study Herpesviruses were not useful—at least not yet. "These studies suggest," they concluded, "that persistence of measles virus in intestinal tissues is a common event and a consistent feature of tissues affected by Crohn's disease."[6]

Two years later, in the first of what would be many scientific refutations of Wakefield's work on IBDs, a group of Japanese researchers from the Akita University School of Medicine wrote a letter to the editor of the *Lancet*. They briefly reported their failure to find evidence that the measles virus was present in the diseased tissues of people with Crohn's disease. The Japanese researchers used the newly developed technique of reverse transcriptase polymerase chain reaction (RT-PCR), which had opened a new realm of exploration for researchers in virology by allowing researchers to search for genetic material from either DNA or RNA. Initially, PCR could be used to detect only those viruses that consisted of DNA, not those consisting of RNA. But many of the viruses of special interest to researchers, such as SARS, influenza, hepatitis C, measles, mumps and rubella, consist of strings of RNA surrounded by a protein shell. To detect the presence of genetic material from RNA viruses, researchers needed to develop a method to reverse engineer RNA back into DNA, then run the PCR technique to quickly copy it many times. RT-PCR allowed them to do just that. So, if the measles virus—either as the wild virus or as the strain used to vaccinate against measles—somehow caused gastrointestinal disorders like Crohn's disease, researchers should be able to find telltale indications of it using RT-PCR on the tissue samples from the intestines of people with the disease, just as they had detected Herpesvirus using PCR.

Encouraged by the Wakefield group's suggestion that Crohn's disease was caused by a persistent infection of the measles virus, another group of Japanese researchers, this one from Hirosaki University School of Medicine, tested for RNA evidence of measles, mumps, and rubella viruses in samples taken from twenty-nine people with Crohn's disease or ulcerative colitis as well as fourteen healthy controls. In 1996, they published a paper in *Gut* reporting that "no measles, mumps, or rubella viral RNA was detected in intestinal tissue from subjects with Crohn's disease, ulcerative colitis, or controls" and that their findings argued "against a persistent measles infection in patients with Crohn's disease." Nonetheless, the paper concluded that despite these negative results, "a continued search for viruses in various areas of the intestine, including the lymph nodes, of patients with Crohn's disease is still justified."[7]

The Wakefield group's 1993 article linking the measles virus with Crohn's disease signaled a shift in the Inflammatory Bowel Disease Study Group's focus. From that point on, first the measles virus and later the MMR vaccine would become the focus of their research as they tried to better understand some of the causes of various forms of IBD. Once they focused on the measles virus as a possible cause of Crohn's disease and other intestinal disorders, the group had to address questions of how and why the virus affected cells in the intestines, when and how the people contracted the virus, and why some people who were exposed to the virus never developed intestinal diseases. In pursuit of these questions, Wakefield and his colleagues employed a number of recently developed research methodologies as well as epidemiological approaches that might help them answer the question of when and how the measles virus might cause or in some way contribute to the development of intestinal disease.

In the early 1990s Wakefield worked with Anders Ekbom, a Swedish physician, and two other researchers to examine the records of children born during measles epidemics in Sweden during the late 1940s and early 1950s. In 1994, they reported they had found that the "number of people with Crohn's disease who had been born after a measles epidemic significantly exceeded that expected," while "the number with ulcerative colitis . . . was close to that expected." They concluded, "Our findings strengthen the hypothesis that measles virus is related causally to Crohn's disease and that the perinatal period could be a time of vulnerability." Two years later, Wakefield, Ekbom, and two other Swedish researchers published another article in the *Lancet* demonstrating a link between measles and Crohn's disease, albeit in a very small number of cases. They had reviewed 25,000 patient files of deliveries that took place during the 1940s at the University Hospital in Uppsala and found four cases in which the mothers had contracted measles during their pregnancy. Of the four children born from these measles-infected mothers, three had been diagnosed with Crohn's disease later in life. "Our study," they concluded, "suggests that exposure to measles virus in utero is a major risk factor for the development of Crohn's disease later in life; such early exposure appears to incur a risk of extensive, aggressive disease."[8]

Wakefield's first published statements about a possible link between measles vaccination and Crohn's disease hint at the MMR-autism furor that he would incite near the end of the decade. In March 1995 Wakefield and Ekbom published "Crohn's Disease: Pathogenesis and Persistent Measles Virus Infection" in the *Journal of Gastroenterology*. They summarized the various evidence that suggested a link between measles and Crohn's disease, and explained that in some countries, such as Scotland, the rate of Crohn's disease increased sharply after the introduction and widespread use of live attenuated measles vaccines in the late 1960s. "If the current upward trend in the incidence of Crohn's disease in children continues and the association holds," they asserted, "the role of vaccination will need to be reviewed." In the concluding section of their paper, they argued that despite the many pieces of evidence suggesting that the measles virus is somehow implicated as a factor in Crohn's disease, "these are not enough." Having established, they believed, a correlation between the measles virus and Crohn's disease, they asserted that much more needed to be done to show how, when, and under what conditions the virus caused or helped cause the disease. In this paper we see Wakefield adopting a rhetorical strategy that he would later exploit to its fullest: allying himself and his work closely with his patients. He and his colleagues concluded, "The tools and techniques necessary to investigate this hypothetical sequence of pathological events are available; whether measles is right or wrong, our long-suffering patients with Crohn's disease deserve an expeditious conclusion."[9]

A month later, in April 1995, the Inflammatory Bowel Disease Study Group directly addressed the possibility that the measles vaccine might be a risk factor for Crohn's disease. They explained that it was reasonable to hypothesize that the "measles vaccination is a risk factor of the development of inflammatory bowel disease," because measles virus infection was found in intestinal tissue using a number of laboratory techniques, because research indicated a strong association between perinatal exposure to measles and the development of Crohn's disease, and because the incidence of IBD in Scotland increased during the same period when use of the live measles vaccine became more routine. They sent questionnaires asking about incidences of particular gastrointestinal diseases to approximately 17,500 people who had been part of long-term follow-up research on the safety and efficacy of measles vaccines. They received completed questionnaires from nearly 15,000 of the research subjects and concluded there was "an association between measles vaccination and inflammatory bowel disease." But they were quick to add, "It does not show a casual relation." Ultimately, however, they asserted that their study provided "further evidence that measles virus has a role in the aetiology of inflammatory bowel disease."[10]

The 1995 paper was the first from the group to generate substantial comment and criticism, and the reaction to it powerfully demonstrated the anxiety that the scientific and medical communities felt about any statement that might undermine the public's trust in vaccines. Recognizing the potential of the paper for controversy, the editors of the *Lancet* commissioned a commentary from Peter Patriarca and Judy Beeler of the Food and Drug Administration's Center for Biologics Evaluation and Research, who asserted that the Wakefield group's paper "leaves a series of troubling questions in its wake." They criticized the manner in which the researchers had recruited their control group as well as how they had interviewed and classified the study subjects. They asserted that Wakefield and his group failed to address why the subjects who had contracted measles had a significantly lower risk of IBD than did those who were vaccinated against it. Despite the limitations that they clearly identified and others that they inferred existed, Patriarca and Beeler agreed that there was a "need for additional studies to confirm whether the association" between inflammatory bowel disease and the measles vaccine "is genuine or spurious"; they also suggested potential paths for that research. They demonstrated their ultimate concern, that scientists, the medical community, or the public at large might conclude from the 1995 paper that vaccines are somehow dangerous or to be avoided. They warned, "We must not lose sight of the frequent and devastating consequences of wild measles virus infection nor forget the millions of lives that have been spared as a result of vaccination."[11]

The following month, the *Lancet* published six letters to the editor, all of which further criticized the Wakefield group's claim that the measles vaccine increased the risk of people developing Crohn's disease. Some of the letters, such as the one jointly written by an employee of the United Kingdom's Statistics Unit of Public Health Laboratory Service and an employee of the Immunisation Division of the Communicable Disease Surveillance Centre in London, argued that the study was flawed because of biases introduced by the "very different methods and rates of follow-up in the two cohorts" studied as well as errors in the questionnaires. Another letter criticized many different methods employed by the group in supporting their hypothesis that the measles virus or the measles vaccine increased the risk of Crohn's disease. They wrote, "Diagnosis based on morphology alone can and has been misleading," and evidence derived from in situ hybridization, immunohistochemistry, and immunogold staining "are all subject to problems of specificity, even in the most careful hands when used at high sensitivity." Other letter writers asserted that the group's epidemiological methods were inappropriate to answer their research questions; instead, they should have employed a case-control study method. K. C. Calman, the Chief Medical Officer for the Department of Health, wrote to inform his colleagues that he had been contacted the prior fall by Wakefield and told about the group's work. Calman was overseeing an aggressive measles, mumps, and rubella immunization campaign, which Wakefield believed was potentially problematic given his group's findings. His "department organized a meeting of independent experts to hear about Wakefield's work and about work that linked Crohn's disease with other infectious agents." They concluded that "there was no indication to recommend changes in existing national immunisation policy and practice."[12]

We see by the mid-1990s, especially in reaction to their 1995 paper in the *Lancet*, that the group had already raised concerns among many members of the British public health community by suggesting that the measles vaccine might play some role in causing Crohn's disease in certain people. The intensity of the response from vaccine advocates demonstrated considerable un-ease among many of the professionals who were responsible for preventing outbreaks of contagious diseases. Calman, the United Kingdom's Chief Medical Officer and among the most ardent supporters of the MMR vaccine when the issue came to a head in 1998, had said three years earlier, "It would be most unfortunate if the publication of this controversial work led to public anxiety over the safety of measles vaccine." Behind the scenes, Calman was in conversation with Wakefield's Dean, Arie Zuckerman, who was "very concerned about the unwelcome controversy surrounding the work on Crohn's disease which is carried out . . . by Dr. Andrew Wakefield and his group." Tony Baxter and John Radford of the Department of Public Health in Doncaster emphasized that "in the interests of broader public health, such investigations should be scientifically rigorous and be designed to answer the question raised."[13]

The clearest indication of the medical community's anxiety over raising public concern about vaccines came with the letter to the editor in the *Lancet* written by six members of the Department of Surgery at St. George's Hospital Medical School in London, who also researched Crohn's disease. The group wrote to refute the Wakefield group's assertion that there might be a causative relationship between the measles vaccine, the MMR vaccine, or the measles virus and Crohn's disease. They pointed out that Crohn's disease emerged twenty years before the introduction of the measles vaccine and that there was no perceivable increase in the incidence of Crohn's disease that mirrored large increases in the rates of measles vaccinations. A newspaper's assertion of a link between measles vaccines and Crohn's disease, and not the scientific paper by the Wakefield group, had motivated them to write. Citing the 1993 *Journal of Virology* paper by the Wakefield group, the letter writers explained, "It has been suggested that the presence of measles virus in the intestine may lead to a granulomatous vasculitis which causes Crohn's disease. A report in *The Guardian* newspaper, November 17, 1993, attributed to the same authors, implicates measles vaccinations as a potential causative factor in Crohn's disease." In similar fashion, an editorial published the following year in the *British Medical Journal* by three public health officials criticized the group's 1997 paper for causing "much parental anxiety" and concluded, "Seeds of concern have been sown among parents and no doubt will continue to be spread. Those advising families must make sure parents can base their decisions on hard science and evidence."[14]

Wakefield and his group fully understood that their work might have implications for the public's support of recommended vaccinations. In their "Authors' Reply" to the letters to the editor of the *Lancet*, they explained, "We reported the measles vaccination study for discussion by the scientific community, not only with many qualifications about its epidemiological aspects but also with great care not to excite media over-reaction. Indeed, we were commended by the U.K. Department of Health for our responsible attitude." Before Wakefield and his colleagues published their controversial 1998 paper that linked the MMR vaccine with gastrointestinal disease and autism, Wakefield and John Walker-Smith had met with several health officials. Overall, the meeting was described as friendly, and the chief medical officer, Calman, agreed to call for a research meeting on the topic, a meeting that never occurred. In contrast to any claims that they acted inappropriately by publishing their findings, Wakefield and his colleagues asserted that it would have been "unethical to suppress this result" simply "because its preliminary conclusions were uncomfortable or inconvenient." More importantly, Wakefield worried that if his group's research was not publicized and it was later learned that the MMR vaccine was in fact responsible for causing either intestinal or development problems, the public's faith in vaccines would be irrevocably damaged. Walker-Smith later explained that Wakefield wished "to avoid a collapse of confidence in immunization as a whole."[15]

The first scientific refutation of the Wakefield group's hypothesis about measles and Crohn's disease came in an early 1996 letter to the editor of the *Lancet*, from the East Dorset Gastroenterology Group. In September 1997, the East Dorset group published the results of their case-control study of 140 subjects which, they concluded, provided "no support for the hypothesis that measles vaccination in childhood predisposes to the later development of either IBD overall or Crohn's disease in particular." In the discussion section of the paper, the authors explained that the vaccine hypothesis had "provoked considerable media interest" that "tended to undermine public confidence about the safety of the highly effective measles vaccine, particularly among parents with IBD who have infants of vaccination age." Their research results, they concluded, showed "no evidence of a link between live attenuated measles vaccination in early childhood and the subsequent risk of developing either Crohn's disease or ulcerative colitis."[16]

Like a production of *West Side Story* cast entirely with English physicians, the East Dorset Gastroenterology Group and Wakefield's Inflammatory

Bowel Disease Study Group faced off in the correspondence section of the December 1997 issue of the *Lancet*. The Wakefield group charged that the East Dorset Group's decisions about which vaccines to include and which to exclude from their study introduced systematic bias into their research and effectively obliterated the evidence of the small number of children who had been harmed by the measles vaccine. The East Dorset Group disputed any claims of systematic bias and concluded that their "finding of no link between measles vaccination and the later development of inflammatory bowel disease is reassuring." Two more gangs of researchers entered the fray: a group of Belgian public health officials and two of the Japanese researchers who had performed the RT-PCR work that refuted the Wakefield group's earlier claims. The Belgians sided with Wakefield by positing what they called the "measles tolerance hypothesis," which suggested that "an association between measles vaccination and Crohn's disease would only be expected in case of vaccination of a child who is (a) not protected by maternal (measles) antibodies anymore, and (b) not yet immunologically mature." The East Dorset Group, the Belgians charged, had not disproven this hypothesis. The Japanese researchers, however, sided with the East Dorset Group by reminding readers of their earlier RT-PCR work; they concluded that their findings were "not in accord with the hypothesis that persistent measles virus infection is the cause of Crohn's disease." The following year, the Wakefield group published similar results when they used RT-PCR and failed to find measles virus RNA in the blood cells or intestinal tissues of patients with IBD.[17]

On the eve of the 1998 publication of the most significant and most contentious paper from the Wakefield group, most of the physicians and researchers who had published on the issue rejected the hypothesis that either the measles virus or the measles vaccine caused IBD. A *British Medical Journal* editorial in January of 1998 declared that the majority of evidence did not "prove a causal link." The World Health Organization's *Weekly Epidemiological Record* summarized the state of knowledge on the possible association between measles infection and the occurrence of chronic inflammatory bowel disease; it declared the notion that "Crohn's disease and other chronic inflammatory illnesses of the intestine might be caused by a virus such as measles" an "interesting hypothesis." It expressed concern about how a "weak epidemiological study," such as the one produced by the Wakefield group in 1993, might "capture media attention" and "cause understandable concern among some parents of children who had received or were about to receive measles vaccine." Ultimately, the editors argued that it would "not be appropriate to alarm recipients of the vaccine by notifying them of this hypothetical risk, thus jeopardizing an immunization programme of proven benefit," and they concluded by quoting the *British Medical Journal's* editor as declaring "the hypothesis dead."[18]

Wakefield's 1998 Paper

Before February 1998, the Wakefield group's suggestions about a potential link between the measles vaccine and inflammatory bowel diseases caused concern only among a relatively small group of medical professionals and received only limited coverage in popular media outlets. This changed when the group published "Ileal-Lymphoid-Nodular Hyperplasia, Non-Specific Colitis, and Pervasive Developmental Disorder in Children" in the February 28, 1998, issue of the *Lancet*. While many papers had been published that had suggested elements of a link between measles, gastrointestinal ailments, and neurological disorders, the 1998 paper was the first to directly connect all three. It described researchers' analysis of twelve children who had been referred to the hospital's pediatric gastroenterology unit for intestinal problems and who all had a "loss of acquired skills, including language." The children underwent thorough medical and psychological examinations, including colonoscopies during which researchers took biopsies of tissues from throughout their gastrointestinal systems. The researchers looked for neurological abnormalities in the children by examining them with magnetic-resonance imaging, electroencephalography, and lumbar punctures. Several of the children drank barium sulfate and their intestines were x-rayed as it traveled through them. Finally, researchers analyzed blood samples drawn from the children. In their paper, the group reported that they found that all twelve children suffered from intestinal abnormalities and had regressive developmental problems, both of which emerged simultaneously.

Given the results of their initial findings on the twelve children, Wakefield believed that it was important for the group to publish their findings quickly, while at the same time continue their research by bringing more children into the study. Everyone directly involved in the research agreed to publish the initial results. Their paper reported that eight of twelve children's parents stated that their child's behavioral problems began shortly after receiving the MMR vaccine. Of the remaining four children, one child's difficulties began after he had contracted measles and another after he had developed an ear infection. All twelve children had intestinal abnormalities, and eleven had patchy chronic inflammation in their colons. The psychiatric evaluations confirmed that nine of the children had autism, one had disintegrative psychosis—also known as Heller's syndrome, a rare condition that causes developmental delays—and two possibly had encephalitis, which is swelling of the brain. The paper identified an association between gastrointestinal disease and developmental regression, and it claimed that both ailments began at approximately the same time and may have been caused by "possible environmental triggers." The group suggested that the trigger was the MMR vaccine.[19]

Thirteen researchers produced the 1998 paper. The diversity of specialists on the team demonstrated the complexity of the research program they had undertaken. Five of them were members of Wakefield's Inflammatory Bowel Disease Study Group, another five worked in the University Departments of Paediatric Gastroenterology. Three other departments—Child and Adolescent Psychiatry, Neurology, and Radiology—contributed one author each. The nature of the research topic required such a broad range of specialists. Wakefield served as the senior scientific investigator and John Walker-Smith was the senior clinical investigator. Simon Murch and Michael Thomson conducted the colonoscopies to take biopsy samples from the children's intestines, which were then analyzed by A. Anthony, A. P. Dhillon, S. E. Davies, and Wakefield. John Linnell examined the children for a vitamin B12 deficiency, because prior studies had suggested that might be involved in neurological disorders. D. M. Casson and M. Malik conducted the clinical assessments on the children, while Mark Berelowitz did the psychiatric assessments, P. Harvey the neurological studies, and A. Valentine the radiological work.[20]

In the discussion section at the end of the paper the researchers explained that the coincidence in the time of onset of the gastrointestinal ailments and the developmental problems, as well as the frequency with which autistic children had intestinal dysfunction, "suggests that the connection is real and reflects a unique disease process." They devoted several paragraphs to explaining the evolution, over the previous three and a half decades and beginning with Hans Asperger's work in 1961, of notions that connected gastrointestinal problems with developmental delays. During the 1970s, Walker-Smith, one of the coauthors of the 1998 Wakefield paper, had identified problems specific to autistic children's intestines. In his memoirs, Walker-Smith explained, "At that time in the late sixties and early seventies, many autistic children had been reported to have bowel problems, and anecdotally there had been reports of benefit from a gluten-free diet." Twenty years later, several researchers posited the "opioid excess" theory of autism, which suggested that "autistic disorders resulted from the incomplete breakdown and excess absorption of gut-derived peptides from foods, including barley, rye, oats, and casein from milk and dairy." The prior research and the group's findings provided the circumstantial evidence they needed to hypothesize that there was a causal relationship between the MMR vaccine, the children's gastrointestinal ailments, and their developmental disorders. Nonetheless, there were still a number of unexplored aspects of the problem, including the question of whether there was a rising incidence of autism after the introduction in 1988 of the MMR vaccine in Britain. Research was needed to better understand why boys were over-represented among people with autism and IBD, why some children seemed to be particularly susceptible, and what role vitamin B12 deficiency (from which most of the children in the research program suffered) played in autism. "Further investigations," they concluded, "are needed to examine this syndrome and its possible relation to this vaccine."[21]

There was significant concern by the editors of the *Lancet* that the authors make clear that their research had not proven a link between the MMR vaccine and autism, but rather had demonstrated a correlation between the two. Following protocol in peer reviewed journals, before publishing the paper, the editor sent it to four anonymous reviewers, all of whom made favorable comments while also posing some questions about the methods used and their interpretation. One reviewer raised what the editor called "a justifiable concern" about the paper's impact "on the public's confidence in a very important vaccine." These comments were all passed to Wakefield, who edited the paper "to make sure it was clear to readers that absolutely no proof existed that the MMR vaccine had caused this strange syndrome." The discussion section of the final version of the paper included a direct statement about the limited nature of the group's claims: "We did not prove an association between measles, mumps, and rubella vaccine and the syndrome described." In the press release by the Royal Free Hospital School of Medicine that preceded the paper's publication, Wakefield likewise stressed that his group had only demonstrated a possible link between the vaccine and autism and that additional research was necessary to better understand the relationship.[22]

By the time the 1998 paper was published, Wakefield had made it difficult for some of his colleagues to continue to support him. Two things in particular stressed their relationships. First, he adopted the position that autism, gastrointestinal disease, and MMR vaccine were all three inextricably linked to one another. Through his nearly decade-long research program, Wakefield came to accept that the proximate cause of autism was an intestinal disorder that prevented children from absorbing or caused them to over-absorb certain foods they consumed. He came to believe that the ultimate cause of autism, however, was the MMR vaccine, which he thought initiated the intestinal disorder. He had significant anecdotal and circumstantial evidence to support individual aspects of his MMR-intestinal-disease-autism hypothesis. Many of his colleagues were willing to support only certain aspects of the work, but not the linked claims that MMR causes intestinal disease, which in turn causes autism.

The second challenge to his colleagues' support came from Wakefield's decision to hold a press conference and publically state that there might be a link between the MMR vaccine, gastrointestinal diseases, and autism. It is not clear who wanted to hold the press conference. Walker-Smith has written that Wakefield and his mentor, Roy Pounder, were "keen" to hold it to discuss the contents of their paper with members of the media. Wakefield contends that his boss and dean of the Royal Free Hospital School of Medicine, Arie Zuckerman, "saw media attention as being a positive thing for a medical school that had been becalmed in the academic doldrums for some years," and that it was Zuckerman who had "made the decision to hold a press briefing on the forthcoming publication, timed for the day before the study appeared in print." Either way, many of the authors of the article refused to attend. According to Walker-Smith, at the press conference Wakefield, "without any evidence, but because of his own fears concerning MMR and his wish to avoid a collapse of confidence in immunization as a whole," recommended that the individual measles, mump, and rubella vaccines be given separately at yearly intervals. Wakefield, however, contends that in fact he had substantial reason for thinking that the combined MMR vaccine was problematic. His 2010 book, *Callous Disregard*, includes the letter that Wakefield wrote to his coauthors explaining the basis for his concerns. "I have thought about this issue almost continuously over the last five years," Wakefield explained. "In addition to our work and that of others, my opinion is also based upon a comprehensive review of all safety studies performed on measles, MR (measles-rubella) and MMR vaccines and re-vaccination policies. This now runs into a report compiled by me of some 250 pages, which I am happy to let you see." In short, based on this evidence, Wakefield believed that by combining three live virus vaccines, the MMR vaccine "has potentially compounded the dangers inherent in the first." He had no doubt, he said, of the value of the continued use of each individual vaccine, but he opposed the combined formulation because of "the risk of apparent synergy between the component viruses."[23]

Knowing the can of worms he was opening by publishing the 1998 Wakefield paper, the editor of the *Lancet*, Richard Horton, took steps to mitigate any controversy that might arise when Britain's premier medical journal published a paper that questioned the safety of one of the most widely used vaccines in the country. In addition to asking Wakefield to state specifically that the group had not proven a causal relationship between the MMR vaccine and autism but only a possible link, Horton also published the Wakefield paper in a section of the journal called "Early Report," to emphasize "the preliminary nature of these findings." Horton included, in the same issue in which the Wakefield paper appeared, two other publications intended as counter-balances to it. The first was a letter from a research group in the University of Edinburgh's Department of Medicine that reported their RT-PCR work examining the potential relationship between inflammatory bowel disease, the measles virus, and measles vaccination. Citing five different papers in which Wakefield was a coauthor, they asserted that RT-PCR was fraught with problems, and that research results from such investigations needed to be carefully considered. "Our experience," they asserted, "demonstrates that even with the most scrupulous attention to methodology and laboratory procedures, cross-contamination of specimens can occasionally occur; and also that considerable experience and a range of methodologies may be needed to recognize non-specific reactions which might be interpreted as positive if confirmatory techniques are not applied." Given this, they concluded from their investigation of nineteen patients with inflammatory bowel disease and eleven control subjects that "measles virus genome is not present in gut mucosal biopsies from patients with Crohn's disease or ulcerative colitis."[24]

Also included in the February 1998 issue of the *Lancet* was a commentary written by Robert Chen and Frank DeStefano of the CDC. Chen and DeStefano framed their discussion around the potential adverse events that Wakefield and his colleagues suggested as being linked to the MMR vaccine. For an adverse event to be accepted as having been caused by a vaccine, laboratory findings and clinical diagnoses must support the claim; these diagnoses can be determined through either a clinical or an epidemiological study.

They explained that epidemiological studies had inherent methodological limitations, so "biological plausibility, consistence, strength, and specificity of association must also be considered in inferring causation." With those provisions established, they asked, "How well then do the features of the association reported by Wakefield and colleagues fit with causality?" Since its inception in the 1960s, hundreds of millions of people, they explained, had been vaccinated with measles-containing vaccine without developing either chronic bowel problems or behavioral problems. They concluded that if the vaccine causes the problems that the Wakefield paper identified, it does so "extremely rarely." Moreover, neither autism nor the intestinal problems that the paper described could be caused solely by the MMR vaccine, because both existed prior to the vaccine. Finally, any potential adverse reactions to a vaccine had to be considered in the context of the tremendous difference between the potential number of cases of a given disease and the adverse events known to be associated with the vaccine for that disease.[25]

In a table of nine different communicable diseases, the highest number of occurrences of each disease in any one year, and the number of adverse events associated with each disease's vaccine in 1997, they showed that there was a drop in incidence of the diseases of between 97.24 percent and 100 percent after the vaccine for each disease was introduced. Chen and DeStefano asked what accounts for the incredibly high number of autistic children with gastrointestinal problems that began shortly after each child's vaccination? They concluded that bias in Wakefield's selection of children and recall bias on the parents' part easily explains it. The last two paragraphs of their commentary made clear the basis for their concern. They described how "vaccine-safety concerns gain prominence whenever the incidence of vaccine-preventable disease fall to negligible levels" and the number of incidents of adverse effects from vaccines rise because of high vaccination rates. Claims like those in the Wakefield paper can "snowball into societal tragedies when the media and the public confuse association with causality and shun immunisation."[26]

Over the next five months, a flurry of letters to the editor were published in the *Lancet* refuting various aspects of the Wakefield group's paper, describing its methodological shortcomings and criticizing the authors or the journal for publishing a paper that could have a catastrophic effect on the public's trust in vaccines. The March 21, 1998, issue of the journal included seven letters, all of which were critical of Wakefield, his colleagues, and their claims. Several letter writers cited previous examples of decline in public confidence in vaccines after reports of problems with particular vaccines were published (such as the vaccine that prevents pertussis). Six public health officials from the Expanded Programme on Immunization at the World Health Organization questioned the merit of publishing the study. Three British public health officials wrote complaining how widely the mass media had reported on the research and how the public concern it had generated was "out of proportion to the strength of the evidence presented." They suggested that it was "time for research publications to carry health warnings so that the public and health professionals are adequately appraised about the strength and quality of the evidence presented." One U.K. physician wrote to protest the publication of the paper because of the "increased credence" Wakefield received by virtue of having his claims published in the *Lancet*. He warned, "I think you will bear a heavy responsibility for acting against the public health interest, which you usually aim to promote." Three researchers from the Scottish Centre for Infection and Environmental Health claimed "that current speculation has undermined confidence in the [MMR] vaccine," and they emphasized researchers' "awesome responsibility" to the public. Two officials from the Institute of Child Health in London claimed that the "only saving grace" for the *Lancet* was "the accompanying well balanced commentary" by Chen and DeStefano.[27]

Wakefield, several of his colleagues, and the editor of the *Lancet* each responded separately to the confrontational letters to the editor. Wakefield wrote one letter and Murch, Thomson, and Walker-Smith wrote another. Wakefield attempted to explain the anger apparent in the letters to the editor from public health officials as evidence of "the rift that can exist between clinical medicine and public health." While public health officials examined the population as a whole, he explained, clinicians are duty-bound to treat individual patients on the basis of information they receive from the patients or the patients' parents. After listening to the parents, he and his colleagues identified a new inflammatory bowel disease that appeared to be associated with his patients' developmental disorders and seemed to arise shortly after the children's MMR vaccinations. Wakefield then went on the attack: "Were we to ignore this because it challenged the public-health dogma on MMR vaccine safety?" Public health officials, Wakefield asserted, "would do well to reflect upon the fact that the published pre-licensure studies of the MMR vaccine safety have been restricted to three weeks." Just as public health officials had used earlier examples to demonstrate the drop in public confidence that followed published reports of vaccine side effects, Wakefield reminded readers that recognition that the pertussis vaccine was associated with chronic neurological disease led to the passing of the Vaccine Damage Payments Act in 1979. He concluded, "Public-health officials would do well to get their own house in order before attacking the position of either clinical researchers or the *Lancet* for what we perceive as our respective duties."[28]

In their separate reply, Murch, Thomson, and Walker-Smith explained that they shared the public health officials' concern about the uptake of the MMR vaccine and explained that they had made clear "both within the paper and forcefully by ourselves at the press conference accompanying the publication" the "absence of hard data supporting the link" between MMR and the intestinal disorders they described. Moreover, they "emphatically endorsed the current vaccination policy until further data are available" and referred readers to newspaper reports about the "sober nature" of their claims at the press conference. They also tried to focus the discussion on what they called "the main thrust of the paper—the detection of a consistent pattern of mucosal abnormality in children within the autism spectrum," which they asserted had been lost in the "emotionally charged debate about the potential role for MMR vaccine in its pathogenesis." This, they asserted, was the paper's most important contribution and one that might allow insights into the causes of and treatments for autism. They concluded, "We suggest that the accompanying commentary was not the only saving grace for *The Lancet*." Walker-Smith explained that from the start he had wanted to avoid any reference to MMR in the paper because he believed that discussing it "might divert attention away from the more important factual results" of the research. He had also refused to attend the press conference that accompanied its publication, explaining, "I do not believe professional research matters should normally be discussed in the public media. They should be discussed in scientific and medical media and at the relevant meetings."[29]

In his reply to the letters, Horton, the editor of the *Lancet*, reiterated the journal's and the authors' emphasis on the preliminary nature of the findings and their multiple references, both in print and aloud, to the fact that they had found no proof of a causal link between the MMR vaccine and autism. He also defended his decision to publish the article, which he said was preferable to "well-meaning censorship," by citing examples of other reasonable hypotheses, such as the recent discovery of a new variant of Creutzfeldt-Jakob disease, commonly known as mad cow disease. Criticism of his decision to publish the Wakefield Group's 1998 paper would follow Horton for years. Ultimately, he viewed the controversy as an example of the difficulties that journal editors faced when they found themselves trying to manage the popular media's reaction to the findings published in professional journals. In response to the letter writers who had attacked him for publishing the paper, Horton countered, "Verification is the right test of new thinking, not censorship." He detected what he termed "a whiff of arrogance" in the debate, as public health officials tried to keep quiet any discussion of possible negative side effects from vaccines. "Can the public not be trusted with a controversial hypothesis?" he asked. "Must people be protected from information judged too sensitive for their consumption by a scientific elite?" Obviously, in a democratic society, the answer was no. He concluded, "If one of the results of freedom of choice is an adverse outcome for the public health, that is a regrettable but necessary consequence of our democracy."[30]

Six weeks later, the May 2, 1998, issue of the *Lancet* offered yet another round of letters, these from critics, supporters, Walker-Smith, Linnell, and two from Wakefield. In addition to reiterating criticisms and defenses, these letters introduced a number of new issues. For the first time, the group's work was attacked by claims that Wakefield had a significant conflict of interest. A letter asserted that it "seems likely" that the children had come to Wakefield's attention by attorneys for the families of children who claimed to be injured by vaccines. In response Wakefield explained that, while he had "agreed to help evaluate a small number of" the children included in the study on behalf of the Legal Aid Board, the children were all referred to him through normal channels. He concluded, "No conflict of interest exists." In his first of two author replies, Wakefield raised the issue of a "possible window-of-opportunity for some children with autism" as justification for his publication of early research results. The window-of-opportunity argument is one that Wakefield and many of his supporters would later use regularly in arguing that early and aggressive intervention with any one of a number of different treatments, ranging from antifungal drugs to radical diets, was justified because doctors had only a limited amount of time to treat certain developmentally delayed children and get them back on track. The letters also included supporting statements from a pediatrician, who confirmed anecdotes about intestinal problems and developmental delays as well as stories about how autistic children improved after their intestinal ailments were treated.[31]

The May 2, 1998, issue of the *Lancet* saw the first contribution from an anti-vaccination activist, Barbara Loe Fisher of the National Vaccine Information Center (NVIC), a Virginia-based nonprofit organization founded in 1982 that claims to be "responsible for launching the vaccine safety and informed consent movement in America in the early 1980s." Fisher is the mother of a child who suffered seizures and swelling of the brain shortly after receiving a DPT injection, and she is the cofounder and president of the NVIC. Fisher defended Wakefield's contentions of a link between MMR and autism and attacked Chen and DeStefano's commentary paper as what she called a "pre-emptive strike by US vaccine policymakers" and an "inappropriate intervention of politics into what should be an apolitical scientific examination." She condemned American public health officials for their unwillingness to accept "any independent thinking or scientific intervention into vaccine-associated health problems that does not carry their imprimatur." While Wakefield found no support for his concern about a possible link between the MMR vaccine, gastrointestinal problems, and autism among the public health community and little support from his colleagues, anti-vaccinationists saw in his work the scientific legitimacy they needed to advance their message about the potential dangers of vaccines to parents and lawmakers.[32]

Wakefield's concern about potential synergistic effects of combining three live vaccines in the MMR vaccine was based in part on some of the research conducted by Scott Montgomery, one of the coauthors of the 1998 *Lancet* paper. In 1995, Montgomery, an epidemiologist in the Social Science Research Unit at City University in London, had performed the statistical analysis that had led to a 1995 paper he cowrote with Wakefield and two others. In "Is Measles Vaccination a Risk Factory of Inflammatory Bowel Disease?" they concluded that "Crohn's disease and ulcerative colitis were reported significantly more often among" people who had received the measles vaccine. The research had caused Wakefield to become concerned about the combined MMR vaccine. In a letter to coauthors prior to that infamous press conference for the 1998 *Lancet* paper, he had cited Montgomery's work in identifying the "apparent synergy between the component viruses" in MMR as a important factor in his recommendation that measles, mumps, and rubella vaccines be administered separately rather than in the combined form.[33]

In 1999, Wakefield and Montgomery published another paper directly asserting a link between the MMR vaccine and autism. They argued that evidence from developed countries indicated that the incidence of autism was rising. "What has changed to cause the sudden and sequential increased risk of this disorder in different countries that use the same diagnostic criteria?" they asked. Genetics alone, the authors argued, cannot account for these rapid increases. Instead, they turned to the "growing concern, among both parents and professionals," that the rapid increase in autism was due to "exposure to the combined measles-mumps-rubella vaccine." The authors then posited that the cause of the apparently increasingly common condition of autistic regression—a condition in which a child develops normally for a time, then loses certain physical or social abilities and regresses into autism— rested on changing patterns of childhood infection. That is, they argued that because of the widespread use of vaccines and the improving material conditions over the course of the twentieth century, children began to be exposed to certain infections, particularly measles, at a different age from when children used to be exposed. Prior to the introduction of vaccination, children encountered most infections in early infancy, and the exposure led to mild fevers and life-long immunities. With improved sanitary conditions, better nutrition, and early childhood vaccination, they asserted, children encountered these infections later in life and as a result the infections were much more dangerous. This was certainly the case with polio, which became a serious public health threat only after material conditions improved and most people were not exposed to it in infancy.[34]

Wakefield and Montgomery used the changing patterns of childhood infection to explain the increasing incidence of autism by asserting that evolutionary history has programmed human immune systems to respond to infections in particular ways at particular ages. Newborns' immune systems, they explained, tend to employ T helper cell type 2 responses to pathogens, while older children's systems tend to use T helper cell type 1 responses to infection. Because of vaccines, they authors posited, modern children confront these infectious agents sometime between the ages of one and three, just as their immune systems are shifting from type 2 to type 1 responses, and their bodies respond by "mounting aberrant immune responses." Such inappropriate immune responses might be triggered or exacerbated by children receiving multiple vaccines at once, as with MMR, and "a close temporal relationship in the exposure of two of these infections during the periods of susceptibility may compound both the risk and severity of autism." Moreover, the immune response might induce multiple ailments in the child, such as gastrointestinal difficulties that accompany or cause developmental difficulties. They termed the combination of gastrointestinal and developmental *autistic enterocolitis.*

Wakefield and Montgomery explained that the syndrome of autistic enterocolitis involved chronic infection of the gut lymphoid tissue; the major symptomatic impact is seen in the child's behavior and development. They explained that there were several "current and by no means mutually exclusive hypotheses for the *liaison dangereuse* between the gut and brain." For example, they described a hypothesis advanced by an American researcher, Vijendra Singh, that autism in some children might be caused by an inappropriate autoimmune reaction that was directed against certain molecules found in nerve cells. Another potential explanation for these children's regression into autism was that a chronic infection of the intestines by a virus or multiple viruses caused a direct toxic effect on the children's developing brains.[35]

For Wakefield and Montgomery, the concept of autistic enterocolitis was not merely a label to apply to a set of symptoms; it was a fundamentally new way to think about both the causes of at least some cases of autism and an approach to treating autistic children. They explained that by accepting their claims that these children's gastrointestinal problems led to their symptoms of autism—rather than the other way around—there were potential therapies that could resolve the children's gastrointestinal ailments and their developmental problems. "In direct contradiction to widely held beliefs in the field of autism," they stated, "there is a reversible element to the behavioral pathology." Citing a 1990 paper from the journal *Brain Dysfunction*, Wakefield and Montgomery asserted, "Dietary exclusion of opioid substrate is one therapeutic approach." The parents of children diagnosed with autism understandably seized on Wakefield's claims about the causes of at least some autistic children's ailments and his offer of a potential cure.[36]

Some support for Wakefield's claims about autistic enterocolitis came in 2000 with a research paper coauthored by six Japanese researchers and Wakefield. The Japanese researchers studied the peripheral blood mononuclear cells (blood cells that are part of the immune system and help fight infection) from forty-eight people, twenty of whom had Crohn's disease, ulcerative colitis, or autistic enterocolitis as it had been defined by Wakefield. Japanese researchers had obtained the nine samples from children with autistic enterocolitis from Wakefield, which is why he was listed as one of the paper's coauthors. Their study used RT-PCR methods to search for sequences of the measles genome in particular blood cells of patients with Crohn's disease, ulcerative colitis, or autistic enterocolitis. The researchers' use of the term *autistic enterocolitis* and, of course, their use of research materials from Wakefield's patients as well as Wakefield's inclusion on the list of authors demonstrates their alliance with him to some degree. The presence of particular RNA molecules in a given sample demonstrated a potential link between the measles virus and the patients' gastrointestinal problems. Prior studies that used the same RT-PCR methods did not show any measles virus RNA in the intestinal tissues of patients with Crohn's disease, but these researchers had looked for it in different regions of the measles virus genome. In the relatively brief discussion section of the paper, the authors concluded that their research suggested that the vaccine strain of measles replicated more quickly than the wild strain. This implied that children who were vaccinated against measles might be more likely to suffer intestinal problems than might those who came to be immune to the measles after they had contracted and recovered from the disease. That same year, however, another group of Japanese researchers using RT-PCR concluded that "there is only a slight possibility that measles virus causes IBD through either persistent infection or molecular mimicry."[37]

From 2000 through 2002, Wakefield worked with a handful of different colleagues to pursue his autistic enterocolitis hypothesis. In June of 2000, he and Montgomery published an editorial in the *American Journal of Gastroenterology* in which they explored the literature on the relationship between the measles virus and inflammatory bowel disease. Again discussing the changing pattern of exposure to an established childhood disease and referencing polio, they concluded that certain bowel diseases probably arise as a delayed effect to "atypical exposure to measles viruses" in combination with factors like genetic susceptibility, age, intensity of exposure, and concurrent infection with other viruses. Three months later, Wakefield coauthored an article in the same journal with eight other researchers, many of whom had been coauthors on the 1998 article that had initiated the MMR/autism controversy. Rather than making any mention of a link between the MMR vaccine and autism, the later article emphasized the issue in which most of the original authors had been most interested: that "a new variant of inflammatory bowel disease is present in this group of children with developmental disorders." An editorial written by two members of the Department of Medicine at the National University of Ireland in the same issue of the journal was generally supportive of the claims from Wakefield's group and congratulated them on "opening yet another window onto the ever-broadening spectrum of gut-brain interactions." They nonetheless cautioned that researchers and clinicians should "resist the temptation to predict causation without the necessary evidence; to do so could engender false hope and further burden families who already have more than their fair share of crosses to bear."[38]

More recently, Wakefield and like-minded figures have worked to distinguish autism as it was described by Kanner in 1943 and as it was canonized in the *Diagnostic and Statistical Manual* in 1980 from a separate, but similarly presenting, ailment called Childhood Disintegrative Disorder (CDD), Heller's syndrome, or disintegrative psychosis. CDD was originally described by Theodore Heller in 1908 as *dementia infantilis* and has only recently been widely recognized. Unlike traditional autism, CDD is characterized by about two years of normal development followed by a period of severe regression and loss of language, play, adaptive, continence, and motor skills. The core symptoms of CDD and autism are the same, but according to Wakefield, children with CDD have normal early development and regression at about two years of age. Because its onset coincides with the barrage of vaccines children normally receive at their second year "well-baby" checkups, it fits nicely into the assertion that a significant number of children categorized as autistic in fact have CDD that is caused or exacerbated by vaccines and perhaps other environmental toxins. Today, most authorities consider regression a feature often found in children diagnosed as autistic, so much so that the common description of autism—such as the one offered by Robert Sears Jr. in *The Autism Book*—asserts that it is generally not the case that "a baby is born with autism and will show signs during the first few months of life." He describes regressive autism alongside early onset autism, halted progression, Asperger's syndrome, and Pervasive Developmental Disorder—Not Otherwise Specified.[39]

Refuting Wakefield

The vast majority of research stimulated by the 1998 Wakefield paper concluded that there was no causal relationship between the MMR vaccine and autism. By the end of 1999, three separate and significant published studies directly refuted Wakefield's assertions.

The first came when several of Wakefield's colleagues at the Royal Free Hospital collaborated with officials from the Immunisation Division of the Public Health Laboratory Service Communicable Disease Surveillance Centre in London to produce a paper for the *Lancet* that pointedly argued against any causal association. The group, led by Brent Taylor, head of the Centre for Community Child Health at the Royal Free Hospital, has become an outspoken critic of Wakefield's work. Their paper detailed their epidemiological study of a potential causal relationship between autism and the MMR vaccine and was directly motivated, they explained, by the previous year's paper from the Wakefield group. They analyzed nearly 500 cases of autism in children born between 1979 and 1998. When they compared children who received the MMR vaccine at a younger age to those who received it later in life, they found no difference in the age of diagnosis. Contrary to Wakefield's reports that parents identified the onset of autism at the time of their MMR vaccination, Taylor's group found no clustering of developmental regression in the months following MMR vaccination. Even more significant was their finding that while there was in fact a steady increase in the number of children diagnosed with autism throughout the 1980s and 1990s, there was no jump in the trend after the introduction of the MMR vaccine in 1988. If Wakefield was correct in his claim that the MMR vaccine in some way caused the symptoms of autism in at least some children, the number of children diagnosed with the problem should have increased substantially after the introduction of the vaccine. Instead, the Taylor group found that there was a steady increase in autism before, during, and after the introduction of the MMR vaccine. Taylor and his colleagues concluded that their research did not "rule out a possibility of a rare idiosyncratic response to MMR," but that nonetheless they could "not support the hypothesis that MMR vaccination is causally related to autism."[40]

As they had done with the Wakefield paper a year earlier, the editors of the *Lancet* included a commentary by DeStefano and Chen in the issue with the paper by Taylor's group. DeStefano and Chen summarized their critique of the earlier Wakefield paper and described the findings from Taylor's group. Throughout the commentary, they emphasized the importance of public confidence in vaccination and criticized the media, which they said had "trumpeted the [Wakefield] study as providing evidence that MMR vaccination may cause IBD." However, just as the Taylor paper had allowed for the possibility of rare cases where the MMR vaccine did trigger or in some way exacerbate developmental problems, DeStefano and Chen stated that there were "cases of regressive disorders for which a biological link with vaccination is plausible," and they cited the 1998 Wakefield paper as evidence.[41]

The second major publication refuting the Wakefield group's claims came from a 1999 report from Britain's Committee on the Safety of Medicine. Experts convened by the Committee on the Safety of Medicines, the Joint Committee on Vaccination and Immunisation, and the Medical Research Council, working with attorneys, sent questionnaires to parents, and reviewed the findings. They concluded that while "it was impossible to prove or refute the suggested associations between MMR vaccine and autism or inflammatory bowel disease," the "information available did not support the suggested causal associations." The report also included a description of a forthcoming paper by the Taylor group and asserted that "parents who have continuing concerns about the safety of MMR vaccine can be reassured," because the vaccine is "the safest way to protect your child."[42]

By 2000, the issue of a possible link between the MMR vaccine and the rapid increase in the number of children diagnosed with autism had ignited concern among American parents and medical professionals. In June 2000, the American Academy of Pediatrics convened a conference of parents, practitioners, and scientists titled "New Challenges in Childhood Immunizations" to discuss research on the MMR vaccine and autism. The paper that resulted summarized the findings by a "multidisciplinary panel of experts" that autism was a complex disorder from uncertain and probably multiple causes. Genetics most likely predisposed some people to developing the condition, and "animal model data support the biologic plausibility that exposure to yet unrecognized infectious or other environmental agents" could cause it. The panel explained that the start of the increase in the number of children diagnosed with autism merely coincided with the adoption of the combined MMR vaccine in the early 1970s, and that epidemiologic studies in Europe indicated no association between MMR and autism. In short, they found no credible research that indicated a link between the MMR vaccine and autism.[43]

In 2001 the British government commissioned a report from the Medical Research Council (MCR), a publicly funded office that distributes research funds, on the state of knowledge about the occurrence and causes of autism spectrum disorders. The report identified gaps in knowledge about autism and sought to "stimulate the research community to develop proposals that address the key issues." Ultimately, the MRC paper relied on the findings from the June 2000 "New Challenges in Childhood Immunizations" conference, concluding that the reports of "immunological abnormalities" have been "many and variable and no conclusive picture emerges, especially as the many confounding factors have been inadequately controlled in the majority of studies." The report devoted several pages to summarizing findings from Britain, North America, and Finland to conclude that the evidence did not support the proposed link of MMR to autism.[44]

By 2002, researchers in several countries had published large-scale epidemiological studies, nearly all of which offered unqualified support for the MMR vaccine and definitively stated that they could not find evidence of a link between autism and the MMR vaccine. Among the most thorough was an article published in *The New England Journal of Medicine* which reported the findings of a study of more than half a million children. The researchers examined the records of all the children born in Denmark from January 1991 to December 1998 to determine if more of the children who received the MMR vaccine were diagnosed with autism than did those who did not receive it. Of the 537,303 children, 738 had been diagnosed with an autism spectrum disorder. The rate of autism was no higher among the vaccinated children. In addition, the researchers found that there was "no temporal clustering of cases of autism at any time after immunization." They concluded that their study provided strong evidence against the hypothesis that MMR vaccination causes autism.[45]

The scientific debate over autism and vaccines ended in the first years of the twenty-first century. Clinical, laboratory, and epidemiological studies all had failed to find evidence of a causal relationship between the MMR vaccine and the symptoms associated with autism. With the exception of an occasional scientific outlaw like Wakefield, no mainstream scientists or orthodox scientific organizations put forward a direct link between the MMR vaccine and autism. By 2002, the scientific controversy over an alleged link between vaccines and autism had ended, but the public controversy had only just begun.

MMR or M, M, and R?

Even before he spoke at the press conference announcing the findings of the 1998 *Lancet* paper, Wakefield pressed medical authorities and public health officials to adopt individual vaccines for measles, mumps, and rubella, rather than giving children the combined MMR. In a February 1998 interview included in a package of resources distributed by the Royal Free Hospital, Wakefield explained that the research that ultimately led him to connect the measles vaccine with autism began about a year earlier, when his group was "contacted by a group of mothers who complained that their children had been developing perfectly normally until they had encountered an environmental insult, [which] in many cases they claimed ... was the measles, mumps and rubella vaccine, and then had lost ... all their acquired skill, such as speech, language, developmental milestones." Wakefield and his colleagues realized that along with the neurological problems, many of the children also had serious gastrointestinal disorders. After examining forty children who had "undergone developmental regression," they found that thirty-nine of them had intestinal ailments that included inflammation of the colon and swollen lymph glands at the end of their intestine.

The interviewer asked Wakefield about the cause of the children's intestinal and neurological problems: "Are you saying now then that there does appear to be a proven link between the vaccine and the side effects?" Wakefield replied, "No, the work certainly raised a question mark over the MMR vaccine," and the group certainly suspected a causal association, but they were far from asserting "a causal assertion that is proven beyond doubt." After being pressed, Wakefield explained that he believed that the Department of Health and Britain's regulatory authorities ought to throw significant resources behind investigations like his and that, in the meantime, the monovalent vaccines—single measles, mumps and rubella vaccines—were likely to be safer than the polyvalent vaccines.[46]

At that time and still today the National Health Service, Britain's publicly funded health care system, does not offer single vaccines against measles, mumps, and rubella. Parents wishing to have their children receive separate vaccinations—or, the "single jab," as the separate vaccines have come to be known in Britain—must use unlicensed vaccines and pay for them themselves. Wakefield's justifications for separating the vaccines are based on his belief that some children's immune systems are overloaded when they have inappropriate reactions to a virus or vaccine. Wakefield and his supporters believe that given all at once, multiple vaccines like the MMR and the new MMRV (measles, mumps, rubella, and varicella) increase the chance that an at-risk child will have a negative reaction to vaccination. By separating the vaccines and allowing the child's body to completely process and recover from each individual vaccine, Wakefield believes, at-risk children would have a greater chance of emerging from the vaccination process unharmed or harmed to a lesser degree.[47]

Health officials in Britain rejected Wakefield's calls to separate the measles, mumps, and rubella vaccines. They argued that separating MMR would cause the "obvious trauma of having three injections instead of one." They also emphasized that by giving the three vaccines at one-year intervals, as Wakefield and his supporters have requested, children will not have full protection against the diseases that are vaccinated against in the second and third years. "This will not only expose the child to the diseases for an unnecessarily long period, but will make it difficult to eliminate them from the population." Finally, health officials have resisted calls to separate the three vaccines because to do so would lend credence to Wakefield's claims. From health officials' all-or-nothing point of view, Wakefield and his supporters were entirely wrong, so it was not appropriate to adopt any portion of their program.[48]

Britain's system of health care providers, which includes both the publicly funded National Health Service (NHS) and private clinics, played a significant role in the debate over the MMR vaccine. The National Health Service provides the combined vaccine to children free of charge, and separate vaccinations for measles, mumps, and rubella are only available through private-pay clinics. Direct Health 2000 is one of the private healthcare groups with clinics in Britain and Ireland that provide single vaccines to paying parents. The company was started by Sarah Dean, a nurse who had worked for several years within the NHS and who believed that it could not always offer the best care available because of "time constraints, no ambition to further develop services, stubbornness to move with inevitable change as well as poor funding." By 2003 there were about three dozen private doctors or clinics offering single vaccines and charging between £60 and £125 (approximately $100 to $200) for each of the three vaccines.[49]

British public health officials responded to the public's interest in single vaccines with statements questioning the safety and efficacy of vaccinating children with individual vaccines rather than the combined MMR. David Salisbury, the Britain's Director of Immunisation at the Department of Health, told the BBC Radio 4's *Today* program that single vaccines were less safe than the combined MMR vaccine for everyone. "If you choose to vaccinate your child with single vaccines you elect to put your child and actually other people's children at risk because you put gaps between the vaccines that are not necessary." Some evidence in support of this claim comes from Japan, the only country where single vaccines are recommended and a country that had regular outbreaks of measles and seventy-nine measles-related deaths in the mid-1990s. Japanese officials had withdrawn the use of the MMR vaccine in 1993 over safety concerns about the use of the Urabe strain of the mumps virus, which was associated with increased rates of aseptic meningitis.

Meanwhile, Irish public health officials emphasized that in Ireland the individual vaccines were not licensed—only the combined MMR vaccine had appropriate oversight. Neville De Souza, the South Eastern Health Board's public health specialist explained, "The single component vaccines are not licensed in this country, so they are not monitored by the Irish medicines Board and their safety, quality and effectiveness cannot be assured." Like Salisbury, De Souza asserted that the delays children experienced between vaccines left them vulnerable for as long as a year to those diseases against which they had not yet been vaccinated. Speaking for Direct Health 2000, Dean responded, "Unfortunately, Irish health officials seem unable to grasp the concept of freedom of choice." Positioning herself as an advocate for parents, she called De Souza's claims that parents might not bother to bring their children back for additional single vaccines "grossly unfair to parents who are not morons and will do the best by their children."[50]

In May 2003, Direct Health 2000 added to the public debate over vaccinating children with individual vaccines rather than the combined MMR vaccine by releasing its analysis of its data. Of the 58,000 children in their records who had received complete courses of the single vaccines, 23,000 of them—nearly 40 percent—had at least one parent who was a health care provider, including physicians and nurses. Dean stated, "These statistics indicate the strong pro-MMR stance adopted by the Health Department is not believed by a large proposition of those who have to promote it." When so many concerned parents are from the medical profession, the perception that the debate about MMR was simply the medical profession versus ignorant parents is weakened. Dean told a *Daily Mail* reporter how a local physician had told her that he "felt extremely guilty" about bringing his son to the clinic on Saturday to receive an individual vaccine "when he had been advising patients to choose the combined MMR jab all week." Kathryn Durnford, a spokesperson for Direct Health, said in February of 2002, "We are now getting as many as 800 calls a day. These are intelligent parents, who feel that the present government policy of offering only the combined vaccination on the N.H.S. does not give them a choice." One of the parents who brought a child to a Direct Health 2000 clinic explained, "I am as concerned as any parent and, of course, I want to protect my baby against major childhood infections, but I am determined to have the choice of single vaccines. I think that three vaccines might be too much for a baby's immune system to cope with."[51]

The British media's relationship to national politics played a significant role in the perpetuation of the public debate over the safety of the combined MMR vaccine. British newspapers leaning in favor of the Labor Party generally supported claims made by government officials and the medical community, while papers favoring the Conservative Party were usually strongly supportive of Wakefield and his claims. The *Daily Mail* and the *Daily Telegraph* both consistently back the Conservative Party as do their readers. They have perpetuated notions that research on the possible link between autism and the MMR vaccine is inconclusive. The *Independent*, however, is a center-left leaning daily newspaper whose readership consists almost entirely of supporters of the Labour and Liberal Democrat parties, and has been critical of Wakefield and his supporters' claims.[52]

Media coverage of the Medical Research Council's 2001 report concluding that there was no evidence linking MMR to autism was similarly skewed. For example, the conservative *Telegraph* headlined its story on the report so as to suggest that the MMR vaccine was still suspected of causing autism: "Studies Fail to Disprove Autism Link with MMR Jab." The article asserted that the "possibility of MMR vaccination causing autism in susceptible children cannot be ruled out on the current evidence," although the link also "has not been proven scientifically." In contrast, BBC News reported that the MRC study backed the safety of the MMR vaccine by ruling "out any link between the MMR vaccine and autism." The MRC study, they reported, "follows numerous others disproving any such link."[53]

Given the charged nature of the issue, it did not take long for elected officials to begin speaking out publicly on what public health authorities believed was a medical, not a political, issue. In January 2001, Julie Kirkbride, a Conservative Member of Parliament and mother of a two-month-old son, accused Britain's health minister of "patronizing bull-headedness" over his steadfast position in favor of the MMR vaccine and against single vaccinations. She fully accepted that there was "no scientific evidence against MMR," but she believed that the choice of single vaccinations rather than the combined MMR vaccine was "a question of a parent's right to choose." Liam Fox, the Shadow Secretary of State for Health (an office held by the opposition party whose job is to scrutinize the actions of the Secretary of State for Health and to develop alternative policies), called for the widespread availability of single vaccines. Access to single vaccines, he maintained, would allow the nation to avoid the threat of a measles outbreak and satisfy the public's anxieties about the MMR vaccine: "It would be better for children to receive a single vaccine than to have nothing at all." Jeremy Laurance, the health editor for *The Independent*, responded to the public pressure for increased access to single vaccines with a long column. "It is not too strong to say," he wrote, "that the views held by Ms. Kirkbride, which are widely shared, threaten a public health disaster."[54]

In December 2001 the public's anxiety over the safety of the MMR vaccine was at the center of a political controversy when Britain's prime minister, Tony Blair, refused to publicly state whether or not his eighteen-month-old son, Leo, had received the combined MMR vaccine. Ian Gibson, the chair of the Commons science and technology select committee and an academic biologist, called for the prime minister and his colleagues to set an example for the public by showing they had vaccinated their children with a vaccine that their government had declared both safe and necessary for the protection of public health. Blair's refusal to confirm that his son had been inoculated with the MMR vaccine led to widespread speculation that the prime minister's wife, Cherie Blair, an advocate of alternative medicine, may have opted for three separate vaccines. Clinics reported being flooded with inquiries from anxious parents about the possibility of their children receiving separate vaccines for measles, mumps, and rubella, which compelled Blair to intimate that his son had received the MMR vaccine: "For the record, Cherie and I both entirely support the advice, as we have consistently said. It is not true that we believe the MMR vaccine to be dangerous or believe that it is better to have separate injects, as has been maliciously suggested in the press, or believe that it is linked to autism." As a political issue, Blair's refusal to comment on his son's vaccination record fueled criticism from the conservative papers that tended to oppose both his Labour Party and the U.K. government's ardent support of the MMR vaccine. The conservative-leaning *Daily Mail* ran six stories throughout mid-December of 2001 pressing for a confession from Blair.[55]

Officials from Britain's medical community were far from sympathetic to Blair's decision to keep his family's medical decisions private. In January 2002, the *British Medical Journal* published a commentary by Caroline White, a freelance medical journalist, that detailed the harm to the public's confidence in MMR that followed Blair's insistence on privacy. White described how conservative-leaning papers used the situation to attack what they viewed as hypocrisy in the Labour Party's position on the safety of the MMR vaccine. The *Daily Mail*, the *Mail on Sunday*, and the *Telegraph* all linked Blair's refusal to state whether his child has received the MMR vaccine to a drop in public uptake of it. Even papers that tended to support the Labour Party and Blair's decision, such as the *Independent*, concluded that his silence on the issue enhanced public doubts about the safety of the combined vaccine. Richard Horton, the editor of the *Lancet*, likewise believed that Blair's refusal to be candid about his family's decision regarding the MMR vaccine "caused thousands of parents to waver once again over vaccinating their children."[56]

In February 2002, amid increasing public concern about the safety of the MMR vaccine and very vocal attacks against him, Andrew Wakefield published a short defense of his work in the *Sunday Herald*. He asserted that the limited amount of research regarding the safety of the MMR vaccine was "totally inadequate from the beginning," and that researchers looked at only "short-term outcomes three or four weeks after vaccination." Throughout the piece, Wakefield emphasized that he was motivated by concerns expressed by parents. "I sit across from you as the parent," he wrote, "and you say: 'this is what happened to my child, they were developing normally, they had speech, language, social skills, they received their MMR vaccine and they developed bowel symptoms and their behavior deteriorated, I lost them, the light went out.'" He asserted that the research he and others performed had shown "that the parents' story is valid. We have found measles virus highly in excess of developmentally normal controls in the diseased (bowel) tissue of children with autism, and not only in the diseased tissue but in the very cells in that diseased tissue that you would anticipate if it were the cause of the disease." Wakefield explained that he is not "inherently anti-vaccine," but that he wants the three vaccines available individually. He concluded by asserting it was not his research that "precipitated this crisis." Instead, it was the "removal of the single vaccine, the removal of choice, and that is what has caused the furor—because the doctors, the gurus, are treating the public as though they are some kind of moronic mass who cannot make an informed decision for themselves."[57]

Marginalized and Radicalized

Late in 2001, Wakefield left his job at the Royal Free Hospital School of Medicine. The *Sunday Times* said his departure was by "mutual agreement," but the *Telegraph* reported that Wakefield had "been forced out of his job" and quoted Wakefield as saying, "I have been asked to go because my research results are unpopular. I did not wish to leave but I have agreed to stand down in the hope that my going will take the political pressure off my colleagues and allow them to get on with the job of looking after the many sick children we have seen. They have not sacked me. They cannot; I have not done anything wrong. I have no intention of stopping my investigations." The *Telegraph* reported that Wakefield resigned his £50,000 a year job because he had been told "that his ideas were 'unwelcome' at University College of London, which controls the Royal Free." By that point, Wakefield claimed to have identified nearly 200 children with a combination of bowel damage and autism after receiving the MMR vaccine. The paper reported, "pressure on the children's gastroenterology unit is so great that its waiting list risks breaking the NHS's eighteen-month limit. Parents have appealed to Tony Blair to give it more funds."[58]

A full six years after the publication of the 1998 *Lancet* article and about two years after Wakefield left the Royal Free Hospital, a freelance journalist named Brian Deer contacted Richard Horton, the editor of the *Lancet,* and asked to meet with his editorial team. He presented to them a "gripping five-hour presentation of the evidence against Wakefield and his colleagues at the Royal Free Hospital," alleging that they had conducted invasive investigations on children without the approval of the hospital's ethics committee, that they had deliberately deceived the ethics committee, that the children in the study had been preselected to insure the desired outcome, and that Wakefield had conducted the study because he had been paid by a law firm that had intended to represent parents who believed that vaccines had harmed their children. The following day, the *Sunday Times* released details of a four-month investigation that claimed to have uncovered "a medical scandal at the heart of the worldwide scare over MMR." Deer reported that "Andrew Wakefield, the doctor who champions the alleged link between measles, mumps and rubella vaccine and autism in young children, stands discredited for misleading his medical colleagues and the *Lancet*, the professional journal that published his findings."[59]

In addition to the apparent bias shown in the reporting of the MMR controversy—with left-leaning papers generally attacking Wakefield and supporting the Labour party, which was then in power, and conservative papers supporting Wakefield's claims and calling for the NHS to start offering individual vaccines—we see the role played by partisanship when Deer brought his allegations to Horton. Deer arrived at the *Lancet*'s editorial offices with Evan Harris, a Liberal Democrat member of Parliament and a physician. In his account of these events, Horton describes how the tension in his meeting with Deer "had been heightened by the shadowy presence of Dr. Evan Harris." After Deer's article appeared Harris called for an independent inquiry into Wakefield's research and, a month later, he stood before the House of Commons and made allegations against Wakefield and his colleagues at the Royal Free Hospital and demanded formal investigations by multiple government agencies.[60]

In response to Deer's accusations, the editors of the *Lancet* drew up and published six specific allegations against Wakefield and his colleagues, all of which were clearly shaped by Deer's reporting. They focused on ethical lapses in acquiring appropriate approval for research and in selecting research subjects, and on Wakefield's potential conflicts of interest. The editors rejected two allegations that the research team had failed to gain appropriate approval from an ethics committee as well as a third allegation that subjects had been selected because they fit the researchers' argument. They concluded, "We do not judge that there was any intention to conceal information or deceive editors, reviewers, or readers about the ethical justification for this work and the nature of patient referral." A statement by the Royal Free and University College Medical School and the Royal Free Hampstead NHS Trust on the matter supported the editors' conclusion that the 1998 paper "had been subjected to appropriate and rigorous ethical scrutiny." However, the editors judged that the last three allegations, all of which focused on Wakefield's failure to disclose potential conflicts of interest before publication of his findings, had merit. Wakefield, they concluded, had received £55,000 from the Legal Aid Board to fund a pilot project to investigate the "grounds for pursuing a multi-party legal action on behalf of parents of allegedly vaccine-damaged children" and "had passed the results of his 1998 paper to lawyers to justify the multi-party legal action." Had Wakefield made this information known to them, they wrote, it would have "been material to our decision-making about the paper's suitability, credibility, and validity for publication." They did not explain how the information would have been used in their deliberations and they failed to offer any conclusions about the paper even after they had that information. In his 2010 book *Callous Disregard*, Wakefield argued that the editors of the *Lancet* had full knowledge of his relationship with the Legal Aid Board but nonetheless claimed that they knew nothing of it before hearing a five-hour private presentation of allegations against Wakefield by Deer. According to Wakefield, Horton used Deer's report as a convenient way to solve the problems created for him and the *Lancet* that were initiated by the 1998 paper. Wakefield claimed that Horton had been under significant pressure from industry, certain elected government officials, and the public health community for his decision to publish the paper, and he alleged that Deer's assertions opened a door for Horton and the *Lancet* to escape through.[61]

In considering sanctions against Wakefield and his coauthors, the *Lancet*'s editors were guided by the Committee on Publication Ethics (COPE), a self-described "forum for editors of peer-reviewed journals to discuss issues related to the integrity of the scientific record." Formed in 1997, one year before Wakefield and his colleagues published their *Lancet* article, COPE provided editors a venue for discussing breaches in research and publication ethics. Following COPE's guidelines, the *Lancet* editors chose to publish the six allegations against Wakefield and his colleagues as well as statements by several of the article's authors. While the allegations centered entirely on the process of researching, writing, and publishing the article, it is clear from the formal statement issued by the *Lancet* that the ongoing public debate about the safety of the MMR vaccine played into their deliberations. They concluded, "Given the public-health importance of MMR vaccination, together with the public interest in this issue, we have decided to pursue a course of full disclosure and transparency concerning these allegations, the authors' responses, the institution's judgment, and our evaluation."[62]

The March 2004 issue of the *Lancet* contained the editor's evaluation of the allegations against the paper as well as statements from Wakefield, Simon Murch, and John Walker-Smith, and it included a retraction by some of the authors. Ten of the original paper's thirteen authors retracted their interpretation of the relationship between enterocolitis and neurological disorders by asserting that they make "no causal link . . . between MMR vaccine and autism" because the data were insufficient. Moreover, because the paper had asserted "the possibility of such a link" and because there had been "major implications for public health," they believed it was appropriate to formally retract their earlier interpretation. Two of the original authors, Andrew Wakefield and Peter Harvey, did not sign the retraction.[63]

While the scientific community and the public grappled with Wakefield's controversial claims, Wakefield grew increasingly aggressive in defending himself and asserting the need to carefully examine the evidence that he and his team had generated. In his response to the first letters to the editor regarding the 1998 *Lancet* paper, Wakefield seemed measured as he focused on issues of method and evidence. By the second round of discussion, which followed the publication of the Taylor group's 1999 paper in the *Lancet*, Wakefield's tone changed considerably. He asserted that "Brent Taylor and colleagues have ignored the rules" of the scientific process by publishing a paper that was "inappropriately didactic." Their methods, he claimed, were weak and their data contradictory. Instead of testing the hypothesis that there is a possible relationship between the MMR vaccine and autism, they "tested the hypothesis that there should be no temporal clustering of first parental concerns with measles, mumps, and rubella vaccination." Wakefield explained that their argument that the increase in autism should, if they were correct, jump immediately after the 1998 introduction of the MMR vaccine into Britain failed to take into account that originally the vaccine was given to all children regardless of whether they had contracted measles before or not. In contrast to the Taylor group's data from London, Wakefield presented data from California that showed a jump in autism rates after the introduction of the MMR vaccine. He defended his work against calls in the *British Medical Journal* and in the "non-peer reviewed so-called analysis in *Current Problems in Pharmacovigilance*" for the termination of research into links between the MMR vaccine and autism. Alluding to his concerns that his critics had abandoned core tenets of the scientific process, Wakefield concluded, "Clearly there are some things that may end-up being terminated as a consequence of these events: research into the possible link between MMR, autism, and bowel disease is not one of them."[64]

Right after the *Lancet* retracted the 1998 paper in 2004, four researchers published "Vaccines for Measles, Mumps, and Rubella in Children," which was a systematic review of the MMR vaccine's effectiveness and side effects as reported in articles published between 1966 and 2004. This was not new re-search and did not examine any new children; rather, it reviewed studies us-ing search words to identify approximately 5,000 articles that contained words like "MMR" or "measles." The researchers whittled the list down to thirty-one articles published between 1971 and 2004 that contained informa-tion on the effectiveness of the MMR vaccine in preventing measles, mumps, or rubella or information on side effects associated with the vaccine. The au-thors devoted most of the discussion and conclusions sections to explaining the obvious effectiveness of the vaccine in eradicating measles and in reduc-ing the incidence of mumps and rubella. Very little space was spent on dis-cussing the most controversial issue related to MMR: Wakefield's assertion that it was linked to increased incidence of gastrointestinal disorders that led to neurological impairment and that children should receive the vaccines in-dividually rather than in a combined form. The authors explained they "found only limited evidence of the safety of MMR compared to its single compo-nent vaccines." They reported that children who received the MMR vaccine had "fewer upper respiratory tract infections, increased febrile convulsions in the first two weeks postvaccination and no increased incidence of aseptic meningitis." They also concluded that their review of existing studies "did not support a causal association with Crohn's disease, ulcerative colitis or autism." The authors did not note that none of the studies under review had set out to examine a relationship between the MMR vaccine, gastrointestinal problems, or neurological damage.[65]

While the review paper said little about its relation to Wakefield's argu-ments, the press release that accompanied the paper's publication made ex-plicit assertions about how the paper directly refuted Wakefield's claims. Just as Wakefield had used a press conference to make claims that went beyond what was directly stated in the 1998 paper in the *Lancet*, the press release that accompanied "Vaccines for Measles, Mumps, and Rubella in Children" ex-tended arguments made in the review article and framed its findings around the MMR debate that Wakefield initiated seven years earlier. The press re-lease asserted that Wakefield's 1998 paper had "triggered a worldwide scare, which in turn resulted in reduced uptake of the vaccine," and it concluded with a list of four "key findings" from the report: there was "no credible link between the MMR vaccine and any long-term disability," the MMR vaccine was a valuable tool in preventing disease, "the lack of confidence in MMR has caused great damage to public health," and "people arguing for or against the use of any therapy need to make sure that they base their conclusions on carefully collected evidence, not just on biased opinion, speculation or suspicion."[66]

The publication of this systematic review incited another round of harsh words from both sides of the MMR debate and perpetuated the public controversy. Wakefield's supporters emphasized the report's concerns that there had not yet been enough study of the efficacy and safety of the MMR vaccine, and they emphasized that the report merely examined published studies rather than directly examining Wakefield's claims. Take, for example, Melanie Phillips, the columnist for the right-leaning *Daily News*, who repeated the review article's claims that the study "had found MMR to be 'safe,' given it the 'all clear' and declared all such fears to be 'unfounded.'" She responded, "This is a load of old baloney," and asserted that "the study didn't say anything like this at all." First, she argued, Wakefield himself "never suggested a link between MMR and Crohn's disease." Instead, he "reported the discovery of an entirely new syndrome, autistic enterocolitis, which produced distressing bowel symptoms along with a number of developmental problems resembling autism," which the review article did not even mention, much less evaluate. She also asserted that despite the claims made in the press release, the report "did *not* conclude that Wakefield's evidence was unreliable." Phillips went on to point out several statements made in the report that were not repeated in the press release, namely, that "the design and reporting of safety outcomes in the MMR vaccine studies, both pre-and post-marketing, are largely inadequate" and that the authors "found only limited evidence of the safety of MMR compared to its single component vaccines." Phillips argued that, far from putting an end to the MMR controversy in Britain, the report and accompanying claims only made worse the "unresolved public health problem." On the other side of the debate, advocates of the MMR vaccine heralded the article for putting to bed the scientific controversy over a potential link between the MMR vaccine and autism. Michael Fitzpatrick wrote in the *British Medical Journal* that the study "confirmed that the scare launched following the now notorious Andrew Wakefield *Lancet* paper in 1998 was finally over." But today, seven years after Fitzpatrick wrote this, British and American parents alike seem as concerned as ever about possible links between vaccines and autism.[67]

After Wakefield left the Royal Free Hospital in 2001, he began working with some U.S. colleagues and supporters to create a research, education, and treatment center for children with autism. With land donated by Tory Ball, a former Dell executive whose son was diagnosed with autism, they opened the Thoughtful House Center for Children in 2005 in Austin, Texas. By 2007 the Thoughtful House had assets of more than $4.5 million and had received donations from individuals, foundations, autism organizations, and corporations, including Ameritrade and the New York Center for Autism. Wakefield served as the center's Executive Director until February 2010.[68]

While Wakefield was in the United States, Britain's General Medical Council began a formal investigation into charges of professional misconduct against Wakefield and two of his coauthors of the 1998 *Lancet* paper, John Walker-Smith and Simon Murch. The investigation was initiated by a complaint by Evan Harris, the Liberal Democrat member of the House of Commons who had accompanied Deer to his first meeting with the editors of the *Lancet*. Wakefield was charged with failing to disclose to the *Lancet* his relationship with solicitors representing parents who believed their children had been harmed by the MMR, for ordering inappropriate medical tests, for failing to disclose how patients were recruited for the study and that some were paid, for performing invasive medical exams without appropriate approval, for conducting a study that was not adequately approved by the hospital's ethics committee, and for paying the parents of some children for blood samples. Wakefield denied the charges and strenuously defended himself. The General Medical Council hearing began in July of 2007. Two and a half years later it concluded that Wakefield was dishonest and irresponsible. In May 2010, he was formally removed from the medical register, and, therefore, is not allowed to practice medicine in the Britain. For his part, Wakefield called the hearing "hypocrisy, double-standards, and professional retribution dressed in sanctimonious piety."[69]

Science and the Celebrity

Concerns about a potential link between vaccines and serious physical or neurological problems had floated around the alternative medicine community throughout most of the 1990s. But it was not until the late 1990s, compelled by the U.S. government-mandated exploration of mercury in food and drugs and Wakefield's 1998 paper, that researchers began a formal investigation of a possible connection between vaccines and the rising number of diagnoses of autism. By 2002, the scientific and medical communities had concluded that there was no relationship between the two and since then have been asserting with confidence that routine childhood immunizations have been scientifically established as safe. Claims to the contrary continue nonetheless and seem to be gaining more support among parents. By 2011, 40 percent of American parents have at some point in their child's lives chosen to delay or refuse a vaccine recommended to them by their pediatrician.

As a parent, I am particularly concerned about the ferocity of the debate over vaccines. Recognizing the need to balance individual liberties with the public good and understanding that, in a liberal democracy, citizens have the right to refuse vaccinations in most cases, I worry about the growing intensity of the debates over vaccines in the last decade because I fear the intensity will drive vaccine proponents and opponents further and further apart. I believe that Wakefield's measles, mumps, and rubella vaccine (MMR)/autism hypothesis is probably wrong, but appreciate his assertion that "the success of vaccination programs requires the willing participation of consumers." It was precisely the same assertion that Robert F. Kennedy Jr. made in his interview with Jon Stewart: "The biggest threat to our vaccine program is that these people have now been caught red-handed conspiring to hide this information from the American people."[1]

Our continuing success in vaccinating children depends on whether the public has confidence in the scientists, doctors, and policy makers (including industry) who shape these programs. It may well be that public confidence is precisely what that small number of ever-present and energized vaccine skeptics, armed with the propagandistic resources of the Internet and granted an audience of vaccine-anxious parents, want to undermine. After all, in any controversy, one of the most effective tools of an insurgency is found in sowing the seeds of doubt and taking advantage of the tentative nature of consensus. Ultimately, however, Wakefield's work was incendiary only because it emerged at a time when so many parents had grown concerned about the modern vaccine schedule and the components of the many vaccines they were compelled allow physicians to give their children. As Richard Horton wrote in the *Guardian*, Wakefield's 1998 paper "fueled a smouldering underground movement against the [MMR] vaccine."[2]

Where does all this leave parents who must make a choice? A recent survey found that 24 percent of Americans believed that because vaccines might cause autism, it was safer not to have children vaccinated at all, and another 19 percent were simply unsure of whether or not vaccines could cause autism. So, a decade after the removal of thimerosal from childhood vaccines and a dozen years after the publication of Wakefield's papers and their rebuttals, nearly half of Americans either believe in or are unsure about a possible link between vaccines and autism.[3]

Speculation about the link extends far beyond the concerns expressed by individual parents; U.S. politicians and celebrities are now questioning the safety of routine childhood vaccines. For example, in February 2008, Senator John McCain, the then-presumptive Republication nominee for president, addressed the issue of a possible link between vaccines and autism at a town hall meeting in Texas. Journalists reported that, in answering a question from the mother of a boy with autism, McCain said, "It's indisputable that [autism] is on the rise amongst children, the question is what's causing it. And we go back and forth and there's strong evidence that indicates that it's got to do with a preservative in vaccines." The editors of the journal *Nature* worried that "such statements have power" and can quickly lead to declining rates of vaccination. They blamed American public health officials for not being more forceful in selling the public on the benefit of vaccinating their children before concluding, "The CDC and other sources of health advice need to be much more sophisticated in how they communicate if vaccination myths are to be successfully countered."[4]

Two months after McCain's statement, the *Washington Post* reported that then-Senator Barack Obama made a similar claim as he campaigned for the Democratic nomination for president. Speaking at a rally in Pennsylvania,

Obama said, "We've seen just a skyrocketing autism rate. Some people are suspicious that it's connected to the vaccines. This person included. The science right now is inconclusive, but we have to research it." A later analysis demonstrated that when Obama said, "this person included," he was referring to the person who had asked a question, not himself, and that Obama believed that vaccinations were necessary to the health of the nation. Nonetheless, Obama's assertion that "the science right now is inconclusive" reinforced the public's concerns about the potential of vaccines to cause autism by suggesting that science had not yet decided the issue. The fact was that the science was far from inconclusive: the medical establishment had concluded that there was no link between vaccines and the onset of symptoms of autism in otherwise healthy children. What is inconclusive is the public discussion on the matter. Attempts to stifle it will drive parents into the arms of people who are unaccredited by the American medical and scientific establishments.[5]

The manner in which the 2008 Republican and Democratic presidential candidates echoed some of the concerns expressed by vaccine-anxious parents mirrors the roles played earlier by Senator Dan Burton and Robert F. Kennedy Jr., in the controversy. It would be difficult to find two more sharply contrasting political ideologies than those carried by Burton and Kennedy; nonetheless, they shared serious concerns about a potential link between vaccines and autism. Their public hearings, statements, and activism did much to broaden discussion of the subject, but neither was able to activate substantial numbers of new followers beyond those who were already engaged. Engaging a wider audience of vaccine-anxious parents required a public figure who could connect to Americans on a personal level and who could engage them in discussions about what they already recognized to be a substantial set of challenges associated with raising children in modern America. These figures begin to emerge in 2007 among a handful of celebrities. The best known of these was a young woman from the Midwest who first came to the public's attention by way of her sex appeal. A decade after her *Playboy* spread, she became an actress and then a mother; subsequently she assumed a new role, as spokesperson for public concerns about vaccines and autism.

Jenny McCarthy and Autism Activism

Jenny McCarthy, the model, actress, and former *Playboy* Playmate of the Year, has emerged as the iconic vaccine-anxious parent and the best-known autism activist of the last several years. Supporters and critics alike frequently hold her up as an example of the modern vaccine-anxious parent, and throughout the last half-decade she has been more celebrated and more attacked than any other figure in this debate. Understanding precisely how she came to play such a central role—and perhaps, more importantly, why she is the iconic vaccine-anxious parent—provides us with some valuable insight into the way in which her opponents and her advocates think about the modern American vaccine debate. The factors that allow her so much appeal to vaccine-anxious parents—her candor, modest background, and girl-next-door appeal—are the same factors that provide her critics with ample ammunition in attacking her concerns.

Born and raised in Chicago in a middle-class family, McCarthy attended Catholic school before studying nursing at Southern Illinois University in Carbondale. While in college, she submitted her picture to *Playboy*, which eventually led to posing in the magazine. She went on to work for MTV and began appearing on sitcoms and feature films while continuing to work with *Playboy*, making public appearances at its events and occasionally posing for magazine shoots. By the mid-1990s she had established herself as a successful model and comic actress.

McCarthy's initial public persona was greatly shaped by her willingness to push social boundaries, particularly those related to sexuality and social convention. One scholar of rhetoric explained, "When Jenny McCarthy posed for a series of Candies shoe advertisements sitting on a toilet with her underwear around her ankles, the taboo nature of the advertisements attracted its fair share of attention, but it also weakened the taboo being violated." Her crass humor has extended into other ads and sketch comedy bits. In the late 1990s, when she began filming her own NBC sitcom, *Jenny,* she struggled to take advantage of her image as sexy boundary-pusher on prime-time network TV. As one trade magazine explained, "And there it is—the looming paradox of McCarthy's move to prime time. How do you market her to the masses without losing that certain Jenny *sais quoi* that got her noticed in the first place?"[6]

In 1999, McCarthy married the actor and director John Mallory Asher and in 2002, their son and McCarthy's only child, Evan, was born. McCarthy and Asher filed for divorce two years later. Beginning late in 2005, she and her son lived with the comedian and actor Jim Carrey. In April of 2010 the two confirmed that they had ended their five-year relationship on good terms.

During the five years with Carrey, McCarthy made the leap from a boorish pin-up girl into the mainstream. She did it not as she had first tried—with movie roles and prime-time TV shows—but by publishing books. McCarthy first tried her hand at writing in 1997 with *Jen-X: Jenny McCarthy's Open Book*, cowritten by Neal Karlen. Published on the eve of her failed sitcom *Jenny*, the book was intended to advance her public image as straight talking, brash, and sexy. Capitalizing on the recent success of books like *The Girlfriend's Guide to Pregnancy*, which offered candid woman-to-woman advice about pregnancy and childbirth, in 2004 McCarthy published *Belly Laughs: The Naked Truth about Pregnancy and Childbirth*, followed by *Baby Laughs: The Naked Truth about the First Year of Motherhood*. These two books vaulted McCarthy's potty humor into the mainstream in a way that a half-dozen B movies and hundreds of celebrity appearances never could. In recent years, other celebrities with public profiles similar to McCarthy's—like Tori Spelling, for example—have followed her example in writing books that demonstrate their evolution from party girl to mother.[7]

McCarthy's fourth book, *Life Laughs: The Naked Truth about Motherhood, Marriage, and Moving On*, was written during the tumultuous year when she divorced her husband and when her son, Evan, was diagnosed with autism. Published in 2006, it was dedicated to "those days when we wake up late for work, feeling fat, gossiped about, screamed at by our children, and not fully adored and nurtured by our horny men." Referring generically to husbands as "Mr. Potato Head," in pithy, two- and three-page chapters, McCarthy discusses trading sexual favors for housework, complains about the tendency of marriage to kill romance, and describes the end of her marriage to Asher. In *Louder Than Words: A Mother's Journey in Healing Autism*, published a year later, McCarthy offered a fundamentally more mature glimpse of herself, the challenges she faced during and after her divorce, and the reality of being the parent of a child diagnosed with autism. It embraced her relationship with the emerging community of parents of autistic children and represents the third stage in her transformation from playmate to mother to activist.[8]

In *Louder Than Words*, McCarthy describes her personal struggles with Asher in parallel with her growing conflict with her son's doctors, all in the context of Evan's diagnosis with autism. Its dedication was a touching tribute to her son, and its contents were in sharp contrast to her earlier books. It begins, as many books and articles on autism begin, with a detailed description of the day Evan's symptoms of autism first appeared. McCarthy found her two-year-old in his crib, limp and struggling to breathe while he had a seizure. She called 911, and an ambulance took him to the hospital where he was given a series of tests and released the next day. When he left the hospital he was unable to walk, barely spoke, and acted oddly, and health care providers could not tell her why. Her discussion of that horrible day is laced with small details that foreshadow her eventual disgust with the medical profession, from the paramedics who had casually walked up her driveway ("I ran outside and screamed, 'Don't fucking walk. Get over here, run!'") to frustration with the glacial pace of hospitals and their bureaucracy ("I learned that 'soon' on hospital terms can mean 'on the next shift change.'") to the doctor she called "a young Doogie Howser neurologist," who dismissed Evan's seizure as an unexplainable one-time event ("I stood there in shock and silence because I couldn't think of a polite way to say, 'You're a fucking idiot.'"). Unable to find solutions to—or even adequate explanations for—Evan's seizure or the radical changes to his physical and cognitive abilities that followed, McCarthy writes that she turned to the Internet: "I decided to start doing some research—and by research, I mean Google. By the end of the book, you will see that I should have a doctorate in Google research, what with all the time I spent online trying desperately to understand what was happening to my baby."[9]

McCarthy—like many other concerned parents—learned a great deal through her Internet research and through a variety of books from her local bookstore. Laypersons' ability to sidestep accredited medical authorities through the Internet and other such non-peer-reviewed publications concerns public health officials. As far back as the late 1990s, physicians and scientists worried about the web's capacity to generate and spread information about vaccines that they did not accept as accurate. Mainstream analyses of online content about immunization have shown that, while there was more positive information about vaccines available on the web, the highest viewership went to sources that offered negative content or sources that presented a debate over the safety and effectiveness of vaccines. Officials also worried about the passion shown by vaccine opponents as well as their capacity to attract anxious parents who had "declining awareness of the seriousness of vaccine preventable disease."[10]

McCarthy's frustration with her son's health care providers paralleled her anger with her soon-to-be ex-husband, Asher. In the wake of Evan's first seizure, as they struggled to cope with their changed son, marital tensions heightened. A week after his stay in the hospital, Evan was scheduled for a follow-up visit to what McCarthy described as "the brain-dead neurologist." As she tells it, "We got to the office, and as expected, we waited four hours to see this doctor in whom I had so little confidence. John [Asher] and I fought horribly the whole time. . . . I had so much built-up resentment that I looked at him and said, 'I want you to move out.'" Alone with her son and his new, troubling symptoms, McCarthy faced his diagnosis with autism as a challenge. She turned to books about autism, which gave her the comfort that Asher and the doctors seemed unable or unwilling to provide. "As I read, I started to feel better. Not because I was reading warm and fuzzy stories about autism, but because I was educating myself on every part of the diagnosis. I felt like I was in the driver's seat."[11]

Eventually McCarthy's self-guided research led her to the kind of information that I described earlier in the book: accusations about vaccine-induced ailments, concerns about the contents of vaccines, and assertions that— somehow—vaccines cause the symptoms of autism. She ultimately concluded that Evan's seizures and accompanying changes in his behavior and cognitive abilities were the result of a set of insults that his body endured, including a series of ear infections and their treatment with antibiotics, a severe case of eczema, and his routine childhood vaccines. Evan's body, she believes, was incapable of handling the combined effects of these insults, and his immune system went haywire. His digestive system stopped being able to process certain foods, and this change lead to a toxification of his system, which caused his symptoms. In an interview with a parenting magazine, McCarthy explained, "Looking back, I'd say, 'God, if a kid is having more than seven ear infections in a year and he's got eczema, there are some issues here—his immune system is obviously under attack, and we need to put him in the sensitive category. Let's just delay some of his shots.'" In short, she adopted an explanation that effectively hybridized anti-vaccinators' claims about thimerosal with Wakefield's hypothesis about MMR and autism. Her account of how she came to believe that Evan's symptoms were linked to vaccines is laced with irritation at what she saw as a careless and authoritarian medical community. She tells readers of her memory of Evan's MMR shot:

> The doctor came into the room, and I said to him, "Evan's getting the MMR shot today?"

"Yep, it's that time."

"Does he *have* to have it?" I said.

He stopped and looked at me and said, "Yes, he has to have it."

"Isn't this the autism shot or something like that?" I said.

"NO!" he yelled. "That's all bullshit. There is no correlation between shots and autism at all." Then the nurse handed me papers I had to sign before they gave him the MMR shot, stating that if anything happened to him from the shot, it was no one's fault."[12]

Shortly after Evan was diagnosed with autism, McCarthy read and implemented Lisa S. Lewis's recommendations in her book *Special Diets for Special Kids*. Lewis has a Ph.D. in biological anthropology from New York University and is the mother of a child with autism. She is the cofounder of ANDI, the Autism Network for Dietary Intervention, and is widely cited within both the alternative medical community and the autism activist community. Part cookbook and part medical discourse, *Special Diets for Special Kids* asserts that some children lack the enzymes that are necessary to process gluten and casein, which leads to them having serious neurological deficits. Just like McCarthy and many other parents of children with autism began their books, Lewis begins her book with the story of how her "sweet, blue-eyed little munchkin who loved to cuddle, 'read' books, sing and play with us and the other children at daycare" contracted a series of upper respiratory and ear infections, which were treated with a broad spectrum antibiotic. Soon after, his behavior began to change and his cognitive abilities began to decline. McCarthy found no miracle cures for Evan in making changes to his diet, but she nonetheless asserts, "Dietary intervention can truly help some children with autism, by removing allergens and biologically active peptides thereby reducing the load that an already over-taxed detoxification system must handle."[13]

McCarthy came to believe that her son's physical and cognitive problems were the result of a combination of genetic and environmental factors. The difference between her view and the orthodox one lies in her beliefs about both the environmental triggers and the appropriate therapy for her son's problems. McCarthy believes that Evan was probably born with a weakened immune system, so "getting vaccinated wreaked havoc in his body, and mercury caused damage to the gut (the gut being the home base for your immune system), which caused his inability to process certain proteins, and one could see the result of this damage when he consumed wheat or dairy." McCarthy

found that changes in Evan's diet profoundly improved his behavior and social abilities. "He was in no way cured from autism," she wrote, "but just three
weeks prior, he had been locked in a world of spinning toys and ignoring
people. Now he was actually trying to tell me what he wanted and responding
to people in the room." The obvious improvement in Evan's behavior and
abilities charged McCarthy with an evangelical furor to spread the message
of the therapeutic value of changes in an autistic child's diet and to attack the
medical community for both its stoic promotion of vaccines and its fatalis-
tic attitude toward autism. "Even though his progress made me so happy,"
McCarthy wrote, "I couldn't help but be pissed off that doctors weren't telling
moms to at least try it. They really were against it. My thinking is that if the
diet works on *some* autistic kids, that would link it to vaccines, and God for-
bid that happened. Doctors will never admit it, and it's a useless war to try
and fight."[14]

Through a group of parents of autistic children whom McCarthy eventually met, she was introduced to aggressive alternative therapies for autism,
including chelation, an accepted medical therapy for treating acute toxic
metal poisoning (such as lead or mercury poisoning). McCarthy did not re-
sort to chelation as a therapy for Evan's problems, but she did describe it as
one potentially useful treatment for children suffering from symptoms of autism. Chelating agents—such as dimercaprol, dimercaptosuccinic acid, or
penicillamine—that are injected into the patient, bond with the toxic metal
which can then be excreted from the body. Near the end of the twentieth century, alternative medicine had adopted chelation therapy as a nonstandard
treatment for heart disease and autism. Recent systematic reviews by mainstream researchers have found no benefit from it for heart disease patients
and reject its use in treating autism based on the assertion that the mercury
in thimerosal-containing vaccines has no relation to the onset of symptoms
of autism.

Over the last several years, McCarthy has grown more and more confident
that Evan's cognitive and behavioral problems are rooted in a genetic susceptibility to the contents of the vaccines he received. Some critics of her public
stance on this issue have stated that Evan's symptoms are more consistent
with Landau-Kleffner syndrome, which is characterized by the loss of language abilities that are caused by the damage done by seizures.[15]

McCarthy found tremendous empathy and emotional support—which she
vilified the medical community for not providing her—within the informal

network of parents of children with autism. The contacts she made with other parents of children with autism also introduced her to the community of autism activists. Over the last several years she has worked with various autism groups; she is the official spokesperson for Talk About Curing Autism and a member of the board of Generation Rescue. Generation Rescue was one of the groups that paid for the advertisement in *USA Today* that appeared on the day Annabelle was born claiming a link between vaccines and autism. For several years she was joined in her activism by her then-boyfriend, Jim Carrey. Together, they were prominent members of the community of parents calling for the complete elimination of all mercury from childhood vaccines, and they did a great deal to advance the concerns about vaccines, environmental toxins, and autism among American parents. A magazine for parents of children with autism described them as "the most powerful couple in the autism community." At the same time, they have been sharply criticized by the American medical and scientific communities, who worry about unaccredited celebrities' abilities to shape the concerns and beliefs of hundreds of millions of Americans and who attack McCarthy and Carrey both for apparently ignoring scientific consensus on the subject.[16]

In 2008, McCarthy and Carrey generated substantial media attention for an annual autism awareness march in Washington, DC. What began in 2001 with only 500 people had swelled to over 7,000 with their help. The slogan for the 2008 march was "Green Our Vaccines," which demonstrated nicely the merging of environmental issues with concerns about vaccines. As the group passed the Health and Human Services Building on Independence Avenue, marchers shouted "Too much, too soon!" and some members of the group yelled "Shame on you!" to the employees inside. At the rally that followed the march, McCarthy and Carrey spoke, as did Robert F. Kenney Jr. McCarthy's message then and since has been more nuanced than simply, "vaccines are bad." Instead, she had explained, "Please understand that we are not an anti-vaccine group. We are demanding safe vaccines. We want to reduce the schedule and reduce the toxins. If you ask a parent of an autistic child if they [*sic*] want the measles or the autism, we will stand in line for the fucking measles."[17]

McCarthy wrote two more books after *Louder Than Words*. These books, along with her activism, have solidified her position in the community of parents of autistic children and further publicized her assertion that vaccines are one of the principal causes of autism. In 2008 she published *Mother*

Warriors, which retold in more detail her story and the stories of a number of other women who faced similar struggles in helping their children cope with and overcome the symptoms of autism. A year later she published *Healing and Preventing Autism: A Complete Guide*, with Jerry Kartzinel, a prominent pediatrician who split from mainstream medicine to support claims like those offered by McCarthy and other members of the alternative medicine and autism communities. The book offers a range of explanations and therapies for children with autism and places blame for much of the autism in America on the shoulders of vaccines and their proponents. "Many people ask me if I had to do it all over again, with a new baby, would I vaccinate?" McCarthy wrote, "The answer is no. Hell no." McCarthy and Kartzinel connect vaccine-induced autism to a range of other ailments associated with autoimmune disorders and methylation (a metabolic process that appears related to a number of cognitive disorders, including schizophrenia, bipolar disorder, and autism). Vital to their narrative is the notion of restorative therapies for children suffering with autism—therapies that are linked to stopping and treating the damage that has been done by vaccines. In the introduction to the book, McCarthy announced that by following Kartzinel's protocol, her son has recovered from autism.[18]

On Oprah Winfrey's show in the fall of 2007, McCarthy appeared with Holly Robinson Peete, an actress and the wife of football player Rodney Peete. Both women had children who had been diagnosed with autism, and both saw in vaccines a potential trigger for autism. At one point an audience member asked Peete, "Are immunizations still the focus of the autism community or are there other potential causes being researched, such as preservatives in food, etcetera?" Peete replied, "Immunizations are just one potential contributor or trigger. . . . There are other environmental factors that are being looked at—infertility drugs, labor inducing drugs, Herpesvirus." Another audience member told Peete, "My gut tells me that I shouldn't go with the traditional vaccine schedule, but I don't know how to make the best decision," and she asked Peete, knowing what she knows now, if she would have made a different decision about vaccines. Peete said, "I would wait on MMR until after two or three years or at least have it broken up into three shots." Again showing how issues associated with thimerosal had effectively merged with Wakefield's hypothesis, Peete explained, "The cocktails—MMR, DPT—are the ones with the highest toxicity and may be hard for some children to handle so young all at once." McCarthy's and Peete's appearance on Winfrey's show generated almost 800 comments on the show's website, all of them illustrating both the incredible passion attached to this debate and the broad range of claims made by parents of and advocates for children diagnosed with autism.[19]

McCarthy's influence in this controversy reached an all-time high after she received Winfrey's approval. In the fall of 2008, Oprah's producers asked McCarthy to interview a woman who in the course of giving birth had become infected with flesh-eating bacteria and had to have all of her limbs and several internal organs removed to control the infection. McCarthy spent six hours interviewing the woman. When the show aired, the interview mingled the woman's tragic circumstances and her heroic perseverance with McCarthy's pitch for what she called "mother warriors," women who demonstrate a spirit of willingness to do anything for their children. In the spring of 2009 came the announcement that Winfrey and McCarthy had agreed to continue working together to promote McCarthy's message, beginning with a blog on Winfrey's website. Industry sources speculated that the deal would ultimately lead to a talk show, as it had for others associated with Winfrey.[20]

Commentators on both sides of this debate have written admiringly of McCarthy's ability to be the ideal spokesperson for parents of children with autism. Even those who may be put off by her overt sex appeal, the origins of her fame, or her foul language begrudgingly admit that she has an amazing ability to speak sensibly and compellingly about the issues of autism, vaccines, modern medicine, and the desperate state in which many mothers of autistic children find themselves. "If you needed a woman to bring hope to these mothers," one author admitted, "you could not ask for better casting than Jenny McCarthy." Reporters explain that McCarthy has a "common touch" and that the "foulmouthed comedian from Chicago [is] never far from the surface." Her real appeal, though, is in her representativeness. She has not started a campaign; rather, she has stepped into a void to give voice to millions of Americans who have a tremendous anxiety over the modern vaccine schedule and have found little or no support from science or medicine. She overtly rejects the assured conclusion of scientists and physicians that vaccines have nothing to do with the rapidly increasing diagnoses of autism, asking, "What number does it have to be . . . for people just to start listening to what the mothers of children who have autism have been saying for years?" Epidemiological and case studies are unconvincing to her, and they always will be: "My science is Evan. He's at home. That's my science." As one article about McCarthy concluded, "Such statements could not have won over mothers and found such a ready audience if there weren't many who felt they were hearing someone state what they had long suspected."[21]

Vaccines' Defenders

If McCarthy is the face of the average vaccine-anxious American parent, Paul A. Offit, M.D., is the representative for the scientific and medical communities' assured confidence in vaccines. Offit is a Professor of Pediatrics at the University of Pennsylvania, coinventor of the vaccine against rotavirus, and the Director of the Vaccine Education Center at the Children's Hospital of Philadelphia. Over the last several years, Offit has strongly advocated for universal vaccination, and he has become the principal critic of claims about a causal link between vaccines and autism. His crusade is predicated on his overwhelming faith in vaccines, an autobiographical mythology in which he claims to have decided to become a doctor at age five after seeing a polio ward, and his description about his life-and-death struggle against hate-mongering anti-vaccinators. In his most recent book, *Autism's False Prophets*, and in the interviews he has done in support of it, Offit dramatically portrays the public controversy over vaccines. He tells readers that angry parents have threatened him and his family. Claims like Offit's, coupled with the anti-vaccinationists' stories of crippling disease following routine vaccinations, compose the increasingly chaotic environment in which we expect parents to make reasoned decisions about their children's health.[22]

In 2008, Offit's promotion of vaccines was joined by a sort of anti-Jenny movement among some actresses who jumped into the debate and sided with vaccine proponents. Shortly after the birth of her daughter, Selma Hayek teamed up with Pampers and UNICEF to raise awareness and money for the tetanus vaccine. Kerri Russell and Jennifer Lopez—both of whom had recently given birth—participated in the "Silence the Sounds of Pertussis" campaign to "raise awareness about the importance of booster shots for new parents and people who come in close contact with infants." Marissa Jaret Winokur became an advocate for the HPV vaccine after being diagnosed with cervical cancer. Jennifer Garner became the spokeswoman for the American Lung Association's "Faces of Influenza" education campaign. In their widely publicized and ugly divorce, Charlie Sheen and Denise Richards feuded over—among many other things—vaccination of their two children.[23]

Among Hollywood's vaccine defenders, the actress Amanda Peet has garnered by far the most press. Just as McCarthy became the principal spokeswoman for concerns about vaccines, Peet has stepped forward in support of
the CDC's recommended vaccination schedule. Her campaign began with an
interview that appeared in the August 2008 issue of the parenting magazine
Cookie. In the midst of talking about her shopping habits and efforts to balance the challenges of her career with raising her eighteen-month-old daughter, she spoke seriously about what she said she felt was "among today's
most pressing public-health issues: infant vaccinations." Peet described how
throughout her pregnancy she was regularly on the phone with her brother-
in-law, an infectious disease fellow at the Children's Hospital of Philadelphia.
He eventually put her in contact with his mentor, Paul Offit. Peet said that in
talking with Offit, she was "shocked at the amount of misinformation floating around, particularly in Hollywood." A video on the magazine's website
showed her reiterating the arguments she had heard from Offit about non-
vaccinating parents' complacency toward the tremendous benefits of vaccines, and talking about rumors that commonly circulate regarding vaccines.
She explained that she was not at all worried about potential side effects of
vaccines, but she was deeply concerned about the "growing number of unvaccinated children who are benefiting from the 'shield' created by the inoculated." She concluded, "Frankly, I feel that parents who don't vaccinate their
children are parasites."[24]

Peet's use of the term *parasites* to describe parents who choose not to vaccinate their children set off a firestorm on the Internet. Over the next year
there were more than 680 postings on the publication's discussion board
about the article. They were evenly divided between readers who were out-
raged by her comments and those who were supportive of her position, many
with reservations about her use of the term *parasites*. Peet quickly responded
with an apologetic letter published on the magazine's website. "I believe in
my heart that my use of the word 'parasites' was mean and divisive; I completely understand why it offended some parents, and in particular parents of
children with autism who feel that vaccines caused their illness. For this I am
truly sorry." The apology made up only a small portion of the response—
most of the letter consisted of a defense of the current vaccination schedule
that parroted the most commonly used claims in support of vaccines: "Vast
reductions in immunization will lead to a resurgence of deadly viruses. . . .
It's so hard to appreciate vaccines now that so few children are dying from

preventable diseases today, but that could all change if we're not vigilant." The *Cookie* article's impact was compounded when Peet recorded two public service announcements for the American Academy of Pediatrics and Every Child by Two's campaign, "Vaccinate Your Baby."[25]

To help readers "get up to speed on the vaccine debate," the editors of *Cookie* augmented their original interview with Peet, the many reader comments, and Peet's response with interviews with Offit and Jay Gordon, McCarthy's current pediatrician. Offit ardently defended vaccines as inherently safe and necessary to the health of U.S. children. Gordon argued that some children are genetically predisposed to the neurological problems that we associate with autism, and that environmental toxins like cleaning fluids, pesticides, and vaccines trigger their problems. He concluded by asserting that the "public health benefits of vaccinating are grossly overstated" and that more lives would be saved if medical authorities spent their time "telling people to breastfeed or to quit eating cheese and ice cream." *Cookies* readers were left with two truly incongruent sets of claims and no intermediary to help generate a coherent understanding of the safety and efficacy of vaccines. Moreover, the entire discussion deals with vaccines as a single entity, rather than recognizing that parents can and do pick and choose vaccines based on their concerns about potential side effects as well as about the risk any particular disease represents.[26]

While McCarthy's public advocacy for parents of autistic children has settled into a critique of the various components in vaccines, Peet's promotion of the CDC's vaccination schedule has taken a particularly strategic turn. After Peet's 2008 statement that parents who did not vaccinate their children were parasites, many people attacked her for discussing vaccines without scientific credentials. The following spring, in an interview with the *Stanford Medicine Magazine*, Peet downplayed her own knowledge, saying, "Obviously, I'm not a biochemist—I was even a dismal science student in school—so trying to learn about the ingredients in vaccines is especially difficult. . . . What I really found out is that I have no aptitude for science and that I know nothing." In an interview with ABC's "Good Morning America," Peet said, "Please don't listen to me. Don't listen to actors. Go to the experts." Peet's know-nothing stance allowed her to downplay her own ability to make an informed decision about the safety and efficacy of vaccines—and to drag all other parents who were not scientists along with her. This is precisely what vaccine experts wanted, because it would invest in the experts an unrivaled capacity to make decisions about vaccines for parents and children. Amy Pisani, former executive director of the pro-vaccine organization Every Child by Two, explained that she believed that the issue of vaccines was too important to be left to celebrities: "We don't want it to be a fight between Jenny McCarthy and Amanda Peet. This is between scientists and the public." Offit likewise appreciated Peet's assertions that she is not a scientist and that the public ought not listen to what she has to say on this subject. He called her position "refreshing." The result of such a claim is to say that health professionals alone have the capacity to fully appreciate the risks and benefits of vaccines, and that therefore the rest of us should simply follow their advice.[27]

While public health officials obviously appreciate support from celebrities like Peet and Hayek, they abhor the attention that critics like McCarthy have garnered. Vaccine advocates like Offit believe that in our current culture of celebrity, the public is more likely to listen to celebrities than to researchers. Offit is correct in worrying that people like McCarthy can have an effect on the debate, but he is wrong to imagine that silencing her will effectively end the public debate and calm parents' anxieties about vaccines. Parents are not looking to actresses or models or professional football players' wives for medical advice. The public empathizes with these people because they represent the concerns that average members of the media-consuming public already feel. Rather than serving as role models or even sources of information, these celebrities have become merely the favored spokespersons in the debate.[28]

On what do I base my assertion that celebrity advocates like Peet and McCarthy represent—rather than shape—public opinion on vaccines? First, claims about the impact of celebrities on parents' notions about vaccines are predicated on a belief that parents are inherently ignorant about science and medicine. Second, resistance to the recommended vaccination schedule increases as a parent's educational achievement increases—that is, parents with college degrees and graduate degrees are more likely to be concerned about vaccines than are parents with less education. Third, people will tend to "consume" celebrities and media sources whose social and political views are most like their own. Celebrity spokespeople might provide laypeople with particular language, arguments, or even the willingness to participate in a social movement. They do not, however, create the impetus for participating in a social movement. They provide access to the issues and validation for the concerns that people have about routine childhood immunizations. They are, in short, not the cause of the problem. They are merely a symptom. Ignoring them or attempting to silence them will only drive their claims and parents' vaccine anxiety underground and into the arms of the handful of authors who are the most vocal critics of vaccines.

The Hard Sell

When it comes to the public's health, there exists in the United States a delicate balance of civil liberties, freedom of choice, privacy, and free market capitalism, on the one hand, and the need for the coordinated implementation of expert advice on the other. This balance is weighed, for example, in our abortion laws and practices. We have legalized abortion in the United States, but we also impose certain restrictions on how and when a pregnancy can be terminated. We likewise impose age limits on alcohol and tobacco consumption, and we control how and when it is sold and consumed. We codify behaviors like seat belt or helmet use, and we use the power of the state to quarantine or involuntarily commit citizens who have certain physical or mental illnesses. In doing so, we effectively curtail individual rights in the name of public health. The balancing of individual rights and the public good is obviously necessary in any liberal democracy.

In considering vaccine policies, we must recognize that individual American's rights to privacy, voluntary consent, and personal autonomy need to be similarly weighed against broad public health concerns. The dogmatic rhetoric of the most zealous—and most vocal—vaccine proponents and opponents simply do not allow for that balance. With the lines already drawn in this debate and the arguments already well honed, parents have only the option to subscribe to one side or the other. Unfortunately, neither side seems to satisfy parents' needs and neither side addresses parents' real concerns.

Public health authorities have attempted to tackle the complicated task of balancing individual rights and public good in the context of vaccines many times. In strategizing about how to encourage people to be vaccinated, they frequently invoke the century-old U.S. Supreme Court case of *Jacobson v. Massachusetts* to assert government's power to force citizens to get vaccinated. In 1905, the court decided that it was within the police powers of the state to enact compulsory sterilizations laws, thus affirming the state legislatures that passed laws compelling citizens to receive specific vaccines. The case originated when a man named Henning Jacobson asked to be excused from receiving the smallpox vaccine, even though the town where he lived had ordered all healthy adults to be vaccinated against smallpox or pay a $5 fine. Jacobson did not want to do either, claiming that the statute "abridged his rights as a citizen and deprived him of liberty without due process of law, thus violating his Fourteenth Amendment rights." The court concluded that, unless a person had a medical condition that could be made worse by the vaccine, citizens of states or locales with compulsory vaccination laws had to comply "for the protection of the public health and the public safety, confessedly endangered by the presence of a dangerous disease."[29]

Despite its frequent invocation, *Jacobson v. Massachusetts* provides public health authorities little or no power to coerce citizens to vaccinate their children, especially those citizens who live in the states that allow for philosophical exemptions. In recognizing the centenary of the *Jacobson* decision, legal scholars have recently examined the role of the decision and the evolution of public health and constitutional law over the course of the twentieth century. They found that while the case carried significant influence in the first half of the century, over the last fifty years its authority has waned due to several factors: the U.S. Supreme Court's recognition of the liberties protected by the fourteenth amendment, the social and legal effects of Nazi atrocities committed during World War II, the development of the Nuremberg Code (which established clear standards for voluntary consent in the context of medical care), and especially the emergence of the civil rights movement. Court decisions since *Jacobson* have recognized the importance of individual liberties and have led to further curbs on the power of the state. Simply put, public health officials often overlook that *Jacobson*'s capacity to compel citizens to receive their vaccinations has substantially diminished over the last half-century.[30]

The efficacy of the *Jacobson* decision is further eroded by state legislatures' increasing tendency to expand the allowable criteria for vaccine exemptions. *Jacobson* was predicated on the court's decision that it was within the police powers of the state to adopt compulsory vaccination laws; that is, state legislatures—not public health officials or courts—have the power to decide precisely how, when, and which vaccines its citizens are compelled to receive. That decision also means that state legislatures—again, not public health officials or courts—have the power to decide to allow people easier access to vaccine exemptions. Public health authorities are chagrined that it is increasingly apparent that state legislatures are growing ever more tolerant of parents' philosophical opposition to mandatory vaccines. At a time when the apparent threat of contagious diseases has declined and new vaccines target diseases that many parents find unthreatening, public health officials need more and more potent laws to compel parents to vaccinate their children. But, instead of empowering officials by passing such laws, legislatures seem evermore willing to provide parents even easier access to vaccine exemptions.[31]

Finally, the *Jacobson* decision is largely irrelevant given the nature of many of the newest vaccines as well as those currently in development. Nineteenth-century and early twentieth-century health concerns over diseases like smallpox and diphtheria established public health officials' paradigm for persuading the public to accept vaccines. Parents required relatively little persuasion to take up vaccines against these deadly and highly communicable diseases, and state legislators were willing to empower public health officials with tools to compel unwilling citizens to comply with mandatory vaccine orders. Over the last quarter-century, however, a new cadre of vaccines has been developed that are fundamentally different from their predecessors in that they are not medically essential to preventing the spread of disease. Given their all-or-nothing approach to promoting vaccines, public health officials have adopted and endorsed these new vaccines right alongside earlier, much more necessary, vaccines against deadly and debilitating diseases like diphtheria and polio. Some legal scholars have encouraged the development of a categorical distinction between vaccines that are medically necessary (such as the vaccine against diphtheria) and vaccines that are a practical necessity (like the vaccine against varicella), which would allow parents access to vital vaccines and allow them to make their own decisions about vaccines against less perilous ailments. Unfortunately, as the intensity of the debates over vaccines have increased, public health authorities seem less willing than ever to make such a distinction.[32]

Some scholars have begun questioning what they consider to be an outdated notion of an inherent tension between civil liberties and public health. Instead, they argue that enhanced civil liberties lead to improved public health, at least in underdeveloped countries. This has been most apparent in the context of discussions about HIV/AIDS, where full recognition of human rights leads to decreased HIV infections because it provides people with the disease full access to preventative measures and therapies. Other scholars, like George Annas, take a long-term view on the issue by asserting that when the state compromises civil liberties in the name of health, their efforts often backfire. Writing in the context of post-9/11 fears of terrorist attacks and discussions about bioterrorism, Annas argued that abuses of civil liberties undermine the public's trust, which is a necessary component of any well-functioning public health program. Therefore, any infringement on civil liberties in the name of public health—regardless of the immediate gains that might be recognized—will ultimately result in losses, as the public's trust in health officials declines and the public becomes increasingly resistant to their recommendations.[33]

Accepting that outright legal coercion is at best a limited tool for ensuring high levels of vaccine compliance, public health officials have turned to public education efforts. When they speak openly about popular concerns about vaccines, they emphasize the need for continued education and dialogue, underscoring their belief that parents resist compulsory vaccination only because they are uninformed. Officials believe that if they provide the public with adequate information and a sense of involvement in the decision-making process, nervous parents will be transformed into diehard vaccine advocates. In the 1990s, as public resistance against mandatory vaccination emerged, officials began emphasizing the need to "educate" parents. For example, a 1994 panel of the Institute of Medicine concluded that the federal government and states should "consider cooperating with private health and advocacy groups to educate parents about the benefits, and occasional risks, of vaccination." That same year the Clinton administration was criticized for spending nearly three-quarters of a million dollars to buy equipment to warehouse vaccines to make them more readily available. Critics said that "the money would be better spent on efforts to educate parents." Following recommendations by medical authorities, legislatures in New York and Massachusetts passed laws requiring that summer camps "educate parents about the risks of meningococcal disease and the existence of a vaccine against it."[34]

Public health officials frequently stress the importance of involving citizens in the decision-making process by emphasizing the need for dialogue about vaccine policy. For example, in the wake of the September 2001 terrorist attacks and the anthrax letters, Dr. Anthony S. Fauci, the director of the National Institute of Allergy and Infectious Diseases, called for "open dialogue" about planned preparations to protect the public's health. The public, he said, "should be given an opportunity to hear an open debate" among the public health officials who were invited to speak. However, the public would not be part of this so-called open dialogue. In neither education nor dialogue do public health officials want the public to engage in the decision-making process. Rather, they believe that a properly "educated" parent is one who accepts the recommendations made by public health authorities and that the only people who ought to be involved in the "open dialogue" are public health officials. In short, "open dialogue" means "let us decide," and "educate" means "do what we say." As the environmental ethicist Michael Nelson recently said to me, public input on vaccines seems much like the public hearings that are held on natural resource issues. "It's become a joke," he said, "and we all know it, though some still go through the motions believing they have some sort of impact. So, the system is broadly broken."[35]

From my point of view—as an historian of science, a professor of science policy, and an informed parent—the debates raging about the potential of vaccines to cause autism are worrisome. They concern me because of the threats to my child's health described by polemicists on either side of the debate, and they concern me because of the obvious shortcomings I see in many of the arguments in this debate. On the one hand, anti-vaccinationists assert that by more than tripling the number of mandated vaccinations over the last twenty years, doctors have unwittingly caused a series of serious health problems, most of them neurological and gastrointestinal. On the other hand are the obvious and near universally accepted public health gains provided by vaccines over the last century and the incredible promise of some of the new vaccines that are on the horizon. Caught between the two, I must decide whether or not to have particular vaccines administered to my daughter. As much as I may appreciate open debate in a democratic society, the increasing intensity of this fight leaves me and millions of other American parents simply confused about what to do, threatened by the possibility of millions of unvaccinated children, and unconvinced by the public health community's increasingly aggressive tactics.

6

Getting to the Source of Anxiety

The public controversy about a possible link between vaccines and autism—which I want to again state exists in the face of powerful scientific evidence to the contrary—concerns me. Over the last two decades we have seen a rapid escalation in both the number of vaccines administered to the average U.S. child and the intensity of the standoff between the U.S. medical community and opponents of mandatory vaccination. Parents are caught in the middle of this increasingly passionate debate. Issues involving individual liberties and public health require a subtle balance of competing goals. In this controversy subtlety has been lost, and the battle of harsh words will likely escalate. Peter Hotez, president of the Sabin Vaccine Institute, has said, "If the surgeon general or the secretary of health or the head of the CDC [Centers for Disease Control and Prevention] would come out and make a really strong statement on this, I think the whole thing would go away." In my view, as I hope this book has shown, a "really strong statement" is hardly what is needed, and it certainly would not make the problem disappear. Public health officials, researchers, and physicians must look beyond the vaccines-cause-autism debates to confront the foundational issues causing so many parents such great concerns. What are these issues?[1]

Problems with the modern vaccine schedule have been oversimplified and bundled into the claim that vaccines cause autism as parents' fears have been supported by the views and efforts of anti-vaccinators. Unfortunately, the scientific and medical authorities have been content to wage their battle in support of universal vaccination within the confines of the vaccines-cause-autism claim. It is certainly reasonable for them to do so. The assertion that vaccines do not cause autism (or, we do not see evidence in our studies that vaccines do cause autism) is much more limited, and it allows them to engage in the debate on the basis of their authority in the realm of science and to use their impressive capacity to analyze the problem scientifically. The result is a very public battle that avoids addressing the essential problems with our vaccine regime. Here, then, are some of the underlying problems.

Vaccine Schedules

In Washington, DC, in 2008, Jenny McCarthy led 7,000 demonstrators all chanting "Too many, too soon." By the start of the twenty-first century, a fully vaccinated six-year-old U.S. child received almost three dozen inoculations containing about fifty vaccines against fourteen communicable diseases. This number grows far higher when influenza vaccines are included, because each year's flu vaccine contains at least three different influenza vaccines, and sometimes additional influenza vaccines are recommended, as happened in the 2009–10 influenza season. Over half of these vaccines are given in a child's first eighteen months of life. Again and again throughout their babies' first years of life, many parents watch carefully in the days and weeks that follow each vaccination for adverse effects.

Childbirth and child rearing have become medicalized in the United States. Parents are expected to bring their children into their pediatricians' offices for a series of appointments that are called "well-child visits." These visits happen at regular intervals, typically within the baby's first week and then at one, two, four, six, nine, twelve, fifteen, and eighteen months, and every year after that up to age six. They typically involve a general physical exam, discussions about development and nutrition with the parents, and vaccinations. Most insurance companies fully cover the scheduled well-child visits, and many uninsured children have access to some sort of state-sponsored health care to allow for them. Well-child visits are essential to the modern U.S. immunization schedule because pediatricians' offices have become the location for almost all routine childhood immunizations, and a sick child cannot be vaccinated. To insure that babies receive all of the required and recommended vaccines in the first years of their lives, parents have to be compelled to bring them into the doctor's office when they are healthy enough to be vaccinated.

Unfortunately, the large number of vaccines given in a child's first year, combined with the relative infrequency of well-child visits, means that many children receive multiple vaccinations at key office visits. At the six-month visit, for example, the CDC recommends children be vaccinated against rotavirus, seasonal influenza, diphtheria, tetanus, pertussis, Hib, pneumococcus, and polio. Parents may find themselves leaving their pediatrician's office with a child who has gotten one nasal spray vaccine (against rotavirus), an oral vaccine (against polio), and four shots (seasonal influenza, DTaP, Haemophilus influenzae type B, and pneumococcus), all combined containing as many as ten different vaccines. The number grows even higher when a child misses one or more of the expected well-child visits because of illness or scheduling difficulties, as was the case with Representative Burton's grandson.[2]

One of the public health community's strategies for universal vaccination leads to the vaccines being given long before there is any reasonable risk that a child could actually contract the diseases against which they are being vaccinated. In the case of the hepatitis B vaccine, for example, U.S. children—regardless of their level of risk for contracting the disease—must be vaccinated within the first days or weeks of their life. Why? Because public health officials want to eliminate the disease and, to do this, nearly universal vaccination against hepatitis B is necessary. Millions of parents fail to bring their children to pediatricians' offices, either because they lack adequate health insurance or because they do not see any need to bring healthy children to the doctor's office. Hepatitis B is one of those diseases—like polio—that once no living person has it, will join smallpox on the list of diseases that vaccines have triumphantly exterminated. Unfortunately, our current strategy to achieve universal vaccination against hepatitis B requires that Annabelle and millions of other newborns receive the vaccine within hours of their birth regardless of whether or not they are at any immediate risk for contracting it. The potential of such a strategy for raising alarm among vaccine-anxious parents—and the ammunition it provides anti-vaccinators—is tremendous.

Vaccines as Enhancement Technologies

A substantial part of the problem we have drifted into not just with vaccines but with all drugs, derives from the awkward distinctions we draw between medical *therapies* and medical *enhancements*. Generally speaking, we consider a medical intervention to be therapeutic (to be a therapy) if it attempts to return a patient to health following the diagnosis of a disease, an injury, or some sort of condition that is easily recognized as problematically abnormal. Vaccines are generally classified as *preventative therapies*, because they are given to healthy people in an attempt to preserve health or normalcy by preventing a disease or condition from appearing.

Medical enhancements, however, refer to attempts to overcome normal human limitations by using medical interventions for nontherapeutic purposes. The most notorious human enhancements are in the realm of sports and include steroids, human growth hormones, and supplements like creatine. Lately, nootropics—drugs that improve mental functions like memory, intelligence, motivation, and attention—have come under criticism as a form of human enhancement. If it is ethically problematic for an athlete to use performance-enhancing drugs, it is perhaps equally wrong for someone participating in competitive intellectual activities to use drugs like Ritalin or Adderall to improve their cognitive abilities. Most Americans approve medical interventions for therapeutic ends, but we have significant angst over the use of medical technology for enhancement purposes, either physical or cognitive.[3]

Vaccines tickled the line between therapy and enhancement even before we extended the vaccine regime beyond immediately threatening communicable diseases. They allow us to resist diseases beyond our normal capabilities to do so. We are now so dependent on vaccine technology that without it many of us would not live as long or as healthily as we do. As vaccines are used with increasing frequency to combat a growing list of natural ailments, they are ever more open to being criticized on the grounds that they have become enhancement technologies.

The path from therapy to enhancement is well worn, so it should not come as a surprise that vaccines have followed it. Among the examples of therapies that have become common enhancements is plastic surgery, which was developed to help people who had been burned, had birth defects, or had other disease- or accident-related physical and aesthetic problems. It evolved into nose jobs, breast augmentation, liposuction, and labiaplasty. Long before they were used by athletes to gain weight, size, and strength, steroids were developed to supplement normal hormone levels, to help people overcome injury or disease, and to regain or maintain weight during recuperative periods. Drugs like Adderall were originally created to treat attention deficit hyperactivity disorder and narcolepsy but are now widely used by college students as a study aid. As a prevention against disease, vaccines have been safely ensconced within the realm of preventative therapies, but as new vaccines increasingly allow us to avoid what many parents see as natural aspects of childhood (like contracting the chickenpox) or to avoid the consequences of unprotected sexual activity (as with the long-promised vaccine against HIV/AIDS), we are on the verge of seeing vaccines follow that path from therapy to enhancement.

In the future, we will face even more trouble from the reasonable assertion that vaccines are enhancement technologies and as such are subject to all the criticisms launched against enhancement technologies. A new class of vaccines is emerging that will prevent someone from being capable of getting high from legal and illegal drugs like nicotine, cocaine, methamphetamines, or heroine. Addiction vaccines are being developed as therapies for people who are addicted and want relief from the urges to partake. As with many other therapies-turned-enhancements, the enhancement uses lurk just beneath the surface. Imagine being able to take your child into your pediatrician's office to be vaccinated against addiction to illegal drugs, something that British health ministers have already considered making mandatory. In the 1990s, when addiction vaccines were only theoretically possible, some medical and legal authorities argued that it would be appropriate to add them to the list of mandatory vaccines once they were developed, because addictions are medically classified as diseases. Like smallpox or polio, addictions are essentially communicable because a cluster of addicted people provides the basis for previously unaddicted people to become addicted. Put another way, if no one was addicted to cocaine, there would be no supply of cocaine and no new addicts having access to illegal drugs. Today, as vaccines for the treatment or prevention of certain addictions are under review by the FDA, U.S. law journals publish articles explaining how anti-addiction vaccines could be incorporated into the existing compulsory immunization schedules.[4]

What Is the Goal?

Clustering vaccines around well-child visits represents a practical challenge for vaccine-anxious parents who watch their very young children receive multiple vaccinations and worry about the emergence of adverse side effects. There also exists a much more deeply philosophical challenge to the number of vaccines that we give children. There are a great number of new vaccines on the horizon, and authorities have heralded their potential to allow us to vaccinate larger numbers of people against larger number of diseases. Moreover, recent advances in microbial genetics and immunology have opened the door for another wave of new vaccines. As one researcher noted, "Both infectious and noninfectious diseases are now within the realm of vaccinology." There are now vaccines for twenty-seven different diseases, and the number of diseases, ailments, and even behaviors that can be treated or avoided by vaccines is continuing to grow rapidly. As of January 2009, the U.S. National Institutes of Health were tracking over 650 different active clinical trials of new vaccines. Even the most ardent proponents of widespread vaccination programs must admit that our future holds a number of complicated political, medical, and ethical issues as we invent and mandate more and more vaccines each year.[5]

As it is, over the last twenty years we have doubled the number of diseases against which we vaccinate, and we have tripled the number of inoculations a child receives. How many more vaccines shall we add to the long list of diseases against which we vaccinate? What exactly is our goal here? The complete elimination of all illness? Would such an objective be possible? What would it mean for how we live, how we think about illness, what we expect from our physicians and scientists, and how we deliver health care within a system that already has such gross inequities? Some prominent philosophers and theorists have started thinking about the consequences of our current biotechnological revolution. While some have celebrated the potential of our technology to help us overcome our natural limits, others have described the threat posed by contemporary biotechnology to "alter human nature and thereby move us into a 'posthuman' stage of history." Clearly, these are not simply scientific questions, even if they do have substantial technical components. They require a thoroughgoing analysis by thoughtful, well-trained professionals drawn from a variety of humanistic and scientific disciplines and a careful weighing of our scientific and medical capabilities against other social needs and wants. Unfortunately, we have ignored the difficult questions inherent to biotechnology and have instead engaged in heated arguments around the claim that vaccines cause autism. Thus we have drifted into our current situation.[6]

A Gender Divide

A number of indicators suggest there might be some gender issues at play in modern U.S. tensions over vaccines and the current vaccine schedule. First, even a casual examination of the makeup of the anti-vaccine community demonstrates intense concern among women about vaccines, and at the popular level vaccine anxieties are most frequently presented by women, to women. Certainly, a substantial portion of the gender imbalance is because women take primary responsibility for routine health care and decisions about children's medical care. A 2005 report by the Kaiser Family Foundation found about eight in ten mothers "take on chief responsibility for choosing their children's doctors (79 percent), taking them to appointments (84 percent), and ensuring they receive follow-up care (79 percent)." Disproportionate gender representation is also seen in the children about whom there is so much concern regarding the risk of autism—boys are four to five times more likely than girls to be diagnosed with autism. This gender imbalance means that we frequently see mothers campaigning for their sons, and much more rarely do we see fathers or daughters involved in the debate.[7]

In addition to mothers' shouldering the bulk of responsibility for their families' medical decisions, it may also be the case that, on average, men and women think and act differently about issues of disease. A large and growing body of research has shown that men and women receive different treatment for similar ailments. Some recent literature has demonstrated that this disparity results in part from the different ways in which men and women describe their conditions to physicians and the generally different level of expectations they have for remedying ailments, all of which combine to lead to lower levels of medical intervention on average for women. But there may well be more to it.[8]

It might be that men and women have—or are represented to have—very different notions about the capacity of humans to overcome disease. These potential differences were illustrated nicely in a recent story in the *New York Times* about cryogenics, the low-temperature preservation of people's bodies or brains after death in hopes that one day advanced medicine will be able to revive them. Three times as many men as women pay to have themselves frozen after death. The article focused on the tension between men who intend to be cryogenically preserved and their wives, who find their aspirations after death at best fanciful and at worse insulting. We see that these men who have adopted transhumanist aspirations to use technology to conquer death are often at odds with their wives, who appear much more willing to accept the natural limits and the unavoidable eventuality of death. How might these differences between how the men and women in this story think about life, death, and medical technology—if the differences indeed exist—impact the public's anxieties about vaccines and the conduct of the modern American vaccine controversy? Is the apparently unrelenting effort to add more and more vaccines to the routine schedule a sort of technological hubris, a self-assured component of a transhuman effort to avoid all illness and death?[9]

Putting aside speculation about gender differences, we see that two very different visions for modern medicine are evident in these discussions. The first perspective imagines modern science and medicine as being capable of heroically conquering all ailments, eventually insuring universal health and extending life indefinitely. The other sees science and medicine as, at best, capable of working in concert with the body's natural processes to aid healing, maximize quality of life, and ultimately accept our mortal limitations. The two perspectives demand different approaches to balancing the economic and political demands of science and medicine with the many other human expectations, so there are frequent conflicts when they meet in policy deliberations. These two competing worldviews also think about vaccines in two very different ways—and increasingly the average American is compelled to line up on one side or the other.

The Safety of Vaccines

A vaccine comes to market only after it has undergone a thorough prelicensure testing to establish both its safety and its efficacy. The testing begins with computer modeling of how the vaccine will work, followed by testing on animals. If these tests suggest that a vaccine will be safe and effective, clinical trials proceed to test first the safety of the vaccine, then its efficacy in preventing particular diseases. Clinical trials proceed in three phases. The first phase typically enrolls less than twenty volunteers and looks for common adverse events. Phase two can include several hundred individuals to determine any general side effects that occur after the vaccine is given. Finally, in the third phase, researchers continue to watch for adverse events while they also determine the efficacy of the vaccine in preventing diseases. Once a vaccine is released, its safety cannot be measured directly; instead, as the Centers for Disease Control explains, its safety is estimated by examining the reported number of adverse events, then a formal scientific study is conducted to distinguish between coincidental adverse events and true reactions. "It is rarely possible to say, whether a vaccine caused a specific event," the CDC concludes.[10]

Post-licensure surveillance of vaccines is conducted by the Vaccine Adverse Event Reporting System (VAERS), which is cosponsored by the Food and Drug Administration and the CDC. It collects information provided by patients and physicians about adverse side effects that show up after a patient is vaccinated. Of the ten million vaccinations given each year, VAERS receives about 11,000 reports, 13 percent of which are classified as serious because they are associated with disability, hospitalization, or life-threatening illness. Two percent (220 people) are reports of death. Of the reports received by VAERS, 85 percent to 90 percent describe mild adverse events, like fever, fretfulness, or limited reactions at the injection site. The system also offers a database that researchers can use as an early warning system, as it served for RotaShield when a small number of cases of intussusception appeared among recently vaccinated infants.[11]

Especially considering how intensely health officials rely on VAERS, there are a number of worrisome shortcomings with the system, primary among them concerns about underreporting of adverse events. Officials explain, "'Underreporting' is one of the main limitations of passive surveillance systems, including VAERS." The degree of underreporting is difficult to ascertain. For example, one study estimated that only about 33 percent of the cases of vaccine-associated polio are reported to VAERS, but that over 95 percent of measles, mumps, and rubella vaccine (MMR)-associated thrombocytopenia (low platelet levels) are reported. We also know that newly released vaccines seem to have higher levels of reporting than do vaccines that have been on the market for some time, a phenomenon that has been called the Weber effect. From another perspective, the voluntary basis for reporting adverse effects to VAERS raises significant concern by health officials because plaintiff attorneys have encouraged their clients to file reports in preparation for going to trial. Paul Offit asserted, "Public health officials were disappointed to learn that reports of autism to VAERS weren't coming from parents, doctors, nurses, or nurse practitioners; they were coming from personal-injury lawyers."[12]

Critics of vaccines have long argued that VAERS, by virtue of being a passive surveillance system, is too slow and too inaccurate to depend upon for the safety of the many millions of vaccines we administer each year. Why, given the tremendous health importance of vaccines and the potential damage that can be done by a faulty vaccine, do we rely on a passive surveillance system? The answer is simple: there is no other practical or theoretical way to monitor vaccine safety. By the very nature of vaccines and the functioning of science itself, one cannot say that any vaccine is perfectly safe. That is, we can never rule out with complete confidence the risk of side effects from a vaccine, so there must be in place some sort of continuing surveillance of vaccines as they are administered. Moreover, we must be constantly watchful for the possible future adverse effects of combining vaccines with one another or with some other drug, food, condition, or situation. Short of constantly running and rerunning clinical trials over and over again—something no reasonable person would demand—a passive system is the only method for discovering any long-term adverse effects, and it comes with certain shortcomings. They must be recognized and accepted for what they are.

Vaccine-anxious parents' concerns about the safety of vaccines is based partly on the claim that officials allow vaccines to come to market without adequate testing and, under pressure from lobbyists, too quickly adopt them as part of the vaccine schedule. By moving vaccines too quickly from active investigation in clinic trials into the passive surveillance system, critics worry, short- and long-term side effects are easily overlooked. Recently, this claim has been especially common in the criticisms of Gardasil, the Merck company's vaccine against the Human Papilloma Virus (HPV). Even proponents of the vaccine have expressed these concerns. For example, Diane Harper, an expert on HPV and one of the scientists that Merck employed to conduct the clinical trials of Gardasil, told a reporter recently that she believed that much of the public controversy around the vaccine was the result of a rush to mandate it for very young girls. "It went too fast, it went too fast without any breaks." She believes that Gardasil is safe, but she thought that more time was needed to watch for potential side effects in larger numbers of girls before any consideration should have been given to mandating the vaccine. "The vaccine has not been out long enough for us to have post-marketing surveillance to really understand what all the potential side effects are going to be." It is easy to understand why Merck, after investing so much money in the development of a new vaccine, would want to begin selling it in large quantities as quickly as possible. However, in the context of a public health concern that rests precariously on a willing public's shoulders, corporate profit motives must be tempered by other concerns.[13]

The All-or-Nothing Approach to Vaccination

There is a striking incongruence in the public debates about vaccines: critics attack *particular* vaccines—such as the vaccines against the chickenpox or HPV—and health officials respond with blanket arguments about the vital importance of vaccines *generally*. The approach allows authorities to respond to parents' concerns without addressing them. It is based on the notion—repeatedly expressed—that the decision about the value of a particular vaccine is best left to the officials at the CDC's Advisory Committee on Immunizations Practices.

There are two net effects of this disconnect in the rhetoric over vaccines, both of which are problematic. First, it signals to parents that the vaccine schedule is an all-or-nothing affair. You either accept that the mandated vaccines are all equally valuable and comply with the entire vaccine schedule, or (if you have concerns about one or more vaccines for any reasons) you reject the schedule in its entirety. Nowhere is this as evident as in the response by Paul Offit to the alternative vaccination schedule offered by Robert Sears, popularly known as Dr. Bob. Sears is a member of a family of pediatricians who have published the widely read Sears Parenting Library. In *The Vaccine Book: Making the Right Decision for Your Child*, Sears offered two revised vaccination schedules, one that spread out vaccinations over a longer time period and another that allowed parents to skip the vaccines for milder or lower risk diseases, like hepatitis B and rubella, while maintaining something similar to the recommended vaccination schedule for more problematic diseases, like diphtheria and pneumococcal disease. He also suggested that parents could delay vaccinating their children against diseases like measles, mumps, rubella, and chickenpox until ten years of age, when a blood test would be done to see if the child had acquired natural immunity; only then would a decision be made about whether to vaccinate the child against any or all of these diseases. In an article in the American Academy of Pediatrics' journal *Pediatrics*, Offit took Sears to task for increasing the time during which children would be susceptible to vaccine-preventable diseases. "In an effort to protect children from harm," Offit concluded, "Sears' book will likely put more in harm's way." For the most ardent vaccine proponents, the current vaccine schedule is the only way to vaccinate children, and any deviation from it is a threat to the public health. Offit's article initiated a wave of responses, both within the journal and online, in which authors lined up on either side of the debate and characterized the two pediatricians' dispute in much the same way others had described the stand-off between Jenny McCarthy and Amanda Peet.[14]

The second negative effect of the all-or-nothing approach to vaccination is produced when officials, in promoting the recommended and mandated vaccine schedule against any threat of alteration, make equivalent all of the diseases against which we routinely vaccinate. In this regard, their efforts to get parents to comply with the vaccination schedule effectively holds the chickenpox vaccine equivalent to vaccines against other, much more deadly and debilitating diseases, like diphtheria and pertussis. In their public rhetoric, they disparage anti-vaccinators' claims, asserting that by questioning the need for a vaccine against chickenpox, anti-vaccinators are asking for the return of childhood scourges like polio. In addition to being logically incoherent, this tactic actually empowers the anti-vaccinationists. By making all the vaccines on the schedule of equal importance, anti-vaccinators can sway vaccine-anxious parents over to their side of the debate by taking advantage of the weak basis upon which we vaccinate against diseases like chickenpox. That is, if (as vaccine proponents claim) every vaccine on the schedule is equally vital to the health and well being of children, then parents who have serious reservations about vaccinating their children against a disease that they see as a childhood rite of passage may come to see all the vaccines on the schedule as unnecessary. The bundling of vaccines—such as the combining of the vaccine against chickenpox with the MMR vaccine to create the MMRV—perpetuates the all-or-nothing approach. It also further reduces parental choice and fuels their concerns about the vaccine schedule.

Front Line Warriors: School and Daycare Workers

Short of an extraordinary public health emergency, the likes of which we almost never see, no one can be legally compelled to be vaccinated. However, you may need to be vaccinated if you want to keep your job (as has been the true of members of the military and first responders like police officers and fire fighters) or, absent a medical, religious, or philosophical exemption, if you want to attend a daycare or school. Since the vast majority of U.S. children attend daycare or school, this arrangement means that our current vaccine policy places the duty of policing vaccine compliance on daycare and school administrators and staff. Thus, a parent who—by choice, oversight, or lack of access—has failed to have their child fully vaccinated will be confronted by an administrator or staff member and threatened with the child's expulsion from that daycare or school. Why exactly am I forced to negotiate the details of my daughter's medical records with the receptionist at her daycare? As I explained in the introduction, I have found myself caught between the bureaucratic demands of the Michigan State Health Department and our pediatrician's overbooked schedule, which has led me to take advantage of my state's philosophical exemption to mandatory vaccinations.

In recent years, citing the limitations of the current system, legal and medical authorities have been seeking ways not just to encourage, but to outright force, parents to vaccinate their children. Faced with increasingly popular religious and philosophical exemptions for childhood vaccinations, some officials have become especially aggressive in enforcing compliance. For example, in 2007 Judge C. Philip Nichols Jr. of Prince George's County Circuit Court in Maryland mailed letters to 800 households "strongly recommending that the children be immunized" and threatening fines and jail time if parents refused to comply. Similarly, Alexandra Stewart of the George Washington University Medical Center published an article in 2009 in the *Michigan Law Review* in which she argued that "public-nuisance law may offer a legal mechanism to hold vaccine objectors liable for their actions." Moving from persuading to coercing to compelling compliance with vaccine policy mirrors the broader trend in twentieth-century public health policy where the imminent threat of contagion brought widespread compliance through persuasion alone, whereas more tenuous disease threats required much more aggressive compulsory measures, like fining or jailing parents or preventing them from sending their children to school or daycare.[15]

Squeezing Pediatricians

Pediatricians have discussed ways in which they can press parents to overcome concerns about vaccines and compel them to allow their children to be vaccinated. Over the last several years, they have debated the wisdom of refusing to treat children who are not fully vaccinated. In 2011, the *Chicago Tribune* reported that the Northwestern Children's Practice in Chicago sent letters to parents stating that it would no longer see those children whose parents had chosen to forego any mandated or recommended vaccine. Doctors at the practice based their decision on the assertion that vaccines were both safe and necessary to protect the public health. Scott Goldstein, one of the physicians in the practice, stated, "All of the available research shows that the safest and most effective way to vaccinate children is on the schedule set by the CDC and the American Academy of Pediatrics (AAP). To go against that schedule goes against proven scientific research and puts patients who do follow the schedule at risk." Nationally, between 5 percent and 10 percent of pediatricians had reported discharging families who, despite physicians' recommendations, had refused to allow their children to be fully vaccinated.

The AAP does not think that such efforts are appropriate, and it encourages pediatricians to continue to provide care to children whose parents are unwilling to follow the vaccination schedule. Research published in the AAP's journal *Pediatrics* has demonstrated that continued dialogue between a physician and parent is the most effective way to increase vaccine uptake. While it might seem reasonable to deny access to health care in order to coerce parents into following the routine vaccination schedule, doing so only drives them further from mainstream medicine.[16]

The pressures on pediatricians to fully vaccinate children become even clearer when one realizes that pediatricians make little or no money when they vaccinate their patients, and many actually lose money in the process. A study that appeared in *Pediatrics* in 2009 examined the financial and operating records of about three dozen private medical practices. It reported, "More than one half of the respondents broke even or suffered financial losses from vaccinating patients." The average loss was 7 percent for the practices. The economic burden is made greater because practitioners must keep between $250,000 and $1.9 million tied up in their on-hand inventory of vaccines, a substantial sum for any small business. The price paid by private practices for vaccines varies wildly, and the average reimbursements pediatricians receive from insurance are almost always less than the upper end of that range, which makes it necessary for offices to buy in bulk to keep their costs as low as possible.[17]

To make matters worse, especially in the context of the anxieties that so many parents feel about giving children multiple vaccinations at the same time, insurance companies' vaccine administration fees are not sufficient to cover the overhead associated with administering vaccines unless a child receives two or more inoculations at a single visit. There is, in fact, little or no money to be made by most pediatricians in vaccinating, unless they can give multiple vaccinations in a single visit or they can vaccinate children assembly-line style and spend as little time as possible discussing the benefits and potential adverse side effects of vaccines with parents. The article explains that the counseling time associated with vaccines increases when media coverage of controversial issues, "such as autism," increases, and as one pediatrician commented in a letter to the AAP's journal, *Pediatrics*, "time is often our enemy in general pediatrics"[18]

What are the sources of anxiety for parents as they confront the modern American vaccine controversy? Parents worry about the high number of vaccines that the vaccine schedule prescribes, especially in their children's first year of life. They see that vaccines are increasingly crossing the line from therapies to enhancements, especially the newest vaccines and the addiction vaccines that are on the horizon. Parents frequently express concerns about the increasingly common intrusions of biotechnology into their lives by advocating for lifestyles that they deem "natural." They do not trust the passive surveillance system that is used by public health officials to watch for problematic side effects from vaccines, and they worry about inappropriate corporate influence in the testing and implementation of vaccines. Health officials' all-or-nothing approach to the vaccine schedule makes parents feel disempowered and often resentful of the vaccine schedule, especially when they find themselves negotiating their children's medical care with school and daycare administrators. Finally, the economic realities of the modern American health system prevent pediatricians from devoting the time and resources that are necessary to allay parents' concerns.

Individually, any of these problems can be addressed, and parents often seem willing to overlook them in analogous situations. Combined, the problems represent a serious threat to U.S. parents' willingness to allow their pediatricians to vaccinate their children. The collective weight of the concerns is simply too much for many parents to bear, as evidenced by the high and growing numbers of parents who opt out of one or more vaccines for their children. We may begin to find our way out of the modern American vaccine controversy only by identifying these problems, admitting they are a basis for concern, engaging cooperatively with parents, and directly addressing as many of these problems as possible.

Conclusion

I have concerns about the modern American vaccine schedule, and I am persuaded by some of the evidence launched against the scientific and medical communities. Because of this, I am willing to become a belligerent in the modern American vaccine debate, but not one who lines up on one side or the other. I dismiss the all-or-nothing approach to vaccines that both extremes push on me. As a parent and a scholar who has examined the claims made by the parties in the debate, I hold that all parents need a new way to think about their children's vaccinations.

I do not accept much of what I hear advocated by the alternative health community, the libertarian critics of vaccine policy, or the anti-vaccinators in general. It is foolish to hold up notions of "natural" as being inherently superior to man-made alternatives. I will tell anyone who wants to adopt what they naively imagine to be a holistically natural lifestyle that (thankfully) technology and culture make it impossible to return to the state of nature that was known to our Paleolithic ancestors. We can, at best, justify choices about how we want to live based on a combination of scientific, moral, theological, economic, and political aspirations. I categorically reject as egotistically libertarian any claim that no one has a right to compel us to do anything with our bodies. We live in an interconnected community and are intensely reliant on one another, a situation that forces us to submit to a multitude of concessions as we balance the pragmatic demands of sharing the earth with the rest of humankind. Finally, I reject anti-vaccinators' core assertion that vaccines represent a dangerous insult to our bodies and that we would be better off without them. I believe, as public health authorities claim, that vaccines represent one of the most effective tools in advancing both individuals' health and the public's health.

All that being said, I agree with many of the claims made by critics of the modern vaccine schedule. First, I accept the primacy of an individual's responsibility as a parent in making medical decisions for his or her children. In weighing the benefits and risks associated with vaccines, parents' primary responsibility is to the health and well-being of their children, rather than to the common good. The public and individual benefits cannot be disentangled from one another, of course. But as exemplified by Sybil Carlson, the woman who told the *New York Times* that she refused vaccination because "I refuse to sacrifice my children for the greater good," they are not interchangeable.

I appreciate the willingness of vaccine critics to question the wisdom of blindly following the advice of the priests of modern science and technology. Countless examples of wrong-headed therapies and dangerous drugs should temper our confidence in the current state of medical knowledge and practice. Science and technology allow us tremendous power to improve the human condition, but they alone cannot make us happy, healthy, or good. Science and technology—and their practitioners—necessarily operate within a complex set of social, cultural, political, and economic systems. The claims offered by scientists and physicians must be weighed against a myriad of other, sometimes competing, claims and values. Indeed, science is not enough.

Finally, I see in much of the rhetoric attacking the modern vaccine schedule an underlying frustration with the condition of medical care in the United States today. Overburdened doctors and nurses, crowded waiting rooms, tremendously expensive insurance, massive profits made by pharmaceutical companies, and an elaborate maze of bureaucracy separating ill patients from the people who are expected to help them all have combined to alienate many parents from the medical establishment. Moreover, although medicine is cloaked in altruistic language, it is a business. One need not be a behavioral economist to understand that we can expect certain problems to accompany any profit-making enterprise.

Within this context, we have to admit that the debates over mandatory vaccines and parents' anxieties about them are only partially about science and medicine. Much like recent debates over global climate change, stem cell research, and the teaching of evolution in public schools, the modern American vaccine controversy is a cultural and a political debate. No scientific finding and no agreement among physicians and scientists can possibly bring it to a close. Scientific findings alone cannot end this debate, because the central questions in the debate are inherently political: Who should be vaccinated? Against which diseases? When and why? Who is financially responsible for these preventive measures? How and why should we compensate the unfortunate few who experience adverse effects? Who should make personal medical decisions for individuals not capable of making them for themselves?

What responsibility do individuals have for one another when it comes to issues of public health?

Several of the concerns parents express about the modern vaccine schedule are rooted in decisions that health authorities have made both in crafting vaccine policy and in communicating their recommendations to the public. One example is the all-or-nothing approach common in the public health community's rhetoric about vaccines. Some problems are inherent to the institutional structures that are involved in vaccinating children, such as the economic losses pediatricians face with vaccines because reimbursement rates are simply too low. Other parental concerns are fundamentally beyond the scope of decisions that health authorities, insurance companies, and politicians have made and are instead rooted in the nature of vaccines themselves. Whether we consciously acknowledge it or not, vaccines are increasingly used for medical enhancement. As we add more vaccines to the schedule, these concerns will become a greater burden on our efforts to maintain high levels of vaccine uptake. Regardless of their origins, each of these concerns needs attention from people who can think reasonably and critically about them, people who can clearly articulate the problems and offer potential solutions with all the vigor employed in the rhetoric of the most ardent anti-vaccinators and vaccine proponents.

In this book, I have described a confusing and contentious environment. And yet I feel strongly that, even within this environment, parents must personally accept responsibility to decide deliberately on their children's vaccines—to decide the best course of action for themselves and their children. Over the last twenty years, just as modern vaccine anxieties have emerged, state legislators have loosened requirements related to childhood vaccinations and attendance at schools and daycares. Today, over half of all Americans live in states that allow for philosophical exemptions to mandatory vaccinations—often requiring little more than a parent's signature on an exemption form. Outside of those states, parents with concerns about vaccines should seek out medical providers who can work with them to find alternatives to the routine vaccination schedule or who can allow them access to the medical exemption offered in every state. Like all children's health care decisions, decisions about vaccines are every parent's duty. In my view, ceding that responsibility to someone else—be it a highly qualified healthcare provider or a rabid anti-vaccinator—is an abdication of that duty.

Responsibly engaging in the process of deciding whether or not, how, and when to vaccinate your child requires continuous self-education on the subject, and an earnest search for a variety of trusted resources. Parents should take advantage of the tremendous amount of information available to them from their pediatricians, in bookstores and libraries, and on the Internet from reliable sources. Unfortunately, too many parents feel compelled to seek information about critical health matters only after their children develop symptoms. There is also danger in yielding to what appears to be an innate compulsion to find authoritative sources that confirm your prejudices and desires. To avoid this trap, parents need to draw on their critical abilities to weigh and judge various aspects of controversial issues by reading widely and not settling on only the material that confirms what they may already think. In every such contentious dispute, elements of truth are to be found on both sides of the debate. It is not a matter of deciding which side you want to subscribe to; rather, it is a matter of gleaning whatever you can from all of the belligerents in the vaccination debate and making decisions for yourself.

Throughout the first couple years of childhood, vaccinations are a routine part of almost every encounter a child will have with medical personnel. They begin almost immediately after birth, with the hepatitis B vaccine, and continue through almost every well-baby visit during a child's first two years of life. Unfortunately, doctor's visits are often rushed affairs. Aides, nurses, nurse practitioners, physician assistants, and pediatricians all perform different tasks. Their time is limited because they are under such tight financial constraints. Parents must prepare themselves for the visits and know what specific questions they will ask about the vaccines. For example, which vaccines does the pediatrician's practice recommend? Which particular formulations do they use? What adjutants, preservatives, and other ingredients are in the vaccines? Most practices adhere closely to the routine vaccination schedule, which is easy to find on the CDC's website. Parents can examine the schedule, think about their child's situation, and consider their options. That way, when they decide in favor of or against a vaccine, they are actually making a conscious choice, rather than simply drifting into a decision that has been made by someone else.

Once they have decided the best course of action, parents will probably find that they will have to defend their decisions. Anyone—parent or otherwise—who has confronted the bureaucratic system of health care providers and insurance companies is well aware of the tremendous coercion they wield over the average layperson. A parent who opts for something different than the recommended vaccine schedule is likely to feel at least some of the system's coercive power. For example, at Annabelle's fourth-year well-child checkup, our pediatrician recommended both the seasonal influenza vaccine and the supplementary vaccine against H1N1 (also known as swine flu). I told him that earlier that year both Annabelle and I had physician-confirmed cases of H1N1 and that I had come to the opinion that that particular year's seasonal flu vaccine was of little value given our particular situation. So, I had decided against allowing them to administer either of the flu shots to her. I simply said, "No, I have decided against it." Over the course of the half-hour visit, three health care professionals pressed the vaccines on us, argued with my claim that because we had both had confirmed cases of H1N1 she should not get the vaccine, and made me repeat, "No, I have decided against it" three separate times. These well-meaning professionals were doing their jobs. And I was doing mine as a thoughtful and informed parent.

Standing up for yourself does not mean staking a position and stubbornly sticking to it. Rather, it means thoughtfully considering the evidence and choosing a course of action. If, in conversations with health care providers or others, additional information emerges, parents ought to take time to reconsider their decisions. But they should not make these decisions in the doctor's office. A friend once told me the advice he had given to his children about sex. In deciding when it was time to lose their virginity, he said, "Don't make the decision in the back seat of a car. Think about it beforehand and decide on a plan." I offer the same advice to parents about their children's vaccinations. Do not make the decision in a rushed moment in the doctor's examination room. Take the time before you see a doctor to think about it and make a decision. Then, do not change your mind the moment you are pressured. Later, away from the coercive pressures that plague our relationships with medical providers, reconsider your decision in light of the information that your pediatrician provided you. You may change your mind. Or you may not.

ACKNOWLEDGMENTS

Long before this book went to press, a number of friends and colleagues read and commented on it, and many more helped me think through the issues I confronted in this project. What you see here is shaped by their comments, criticisms, and suggestions, and I sincerely appreciate their work. Among the many people who deserve credit are Matt Zierler, John Waller, Helen Veit, Susan Stein-Roggenbuck, Nathan Praschan, Michael Nelson, Kim Neir, Georgina Montgomery, Yasumasa Komori, Dan Kramer, Benjamin Kleinerman, Dan Kenney, Sally Gregory Kohlstedt, Mott Greene, Melinda Gormley, Waseem El-Rayes, Erik Conway, Kendra Cheruvelil, and Marci Baranski. Tobin Craig deserves special thanks for all the time and attention he has given to this project from start to end. Likewise, I need to single out Audra Wolfe of The Outside Reader and Jackie Wehmueller of the Johns Hopkins University Press, who helped me sharpen the book's argument, clarify my writing, and showed me just how valuable a great editor is.

This book was written during an especially tumultuous time in my life, which I discuss a little in the book's introduction. I would not have survived it without the love and support of my mom, Betty Largent. Likewise, Chris and Nickie Foley stepped into my life just when I most needed them. Eric Berg, my best friend for nearly a quarter of a century, has been a role model for me in both my personal and my professional lives. Over the last several years John Jackson, Michael Reidy, and Jeff Matthews have made regular trips to Michigan to provide camaraderie and to make sure that Annabelle and I stayed on track. Brie Weaver, now Brie Largent, provided me unwavering love and support as this book finally neared completion. Brie, along with Paul, Melanie, and Rachel Weaver, adopted Annabelle and me into their family and provided us a foundation to build a new future together. Finally, I want to thank Chris Young, to whom this book is dedicated. Chris is the truest and most thoughtful friend anyone could have. Thank you all.

Introduction

1. Liz Szabo, "Refusing Kid's Vaccine More Common among Parents," *USA Today,* June 3, 2010.

2. "putchildrenfirst.com," advertisement, *USA Today,* April 6, 2006.

3. Michigan Department of Community Health, "Required Immunizations for Michigan Childcare/Preschool Attendance," www.michigan.gov/documents /PreSchoolRules_170325_7.pdf (accessed December 17, 2008); "Required Immunizations for Michigan School Settings," www.michigan.gov/documents/SchoolRules _170324_7.pdf (accessed December 17, 2008).

4. Centers for Disease Control and Prevention, "CDC Viral Hepatitis," www.cdc .gov/hepatitis/index.htm (accessed December 17, 2008).

5. N. Anthony, M. Reed, A. M. Leff, J. Hugger, and B. Stephens, "Immunization: Public Health Programming through Law Enforcement," *American Journal of Public Health* 67 (1977): 763–64; Jennifer S. Rota, Daniel A. Salmon, Lance E. Rodewald, Robert T. Chen, Beth F. Hibbs, and Eugen J. Gangarosa, "Processes for Obtaining Nonmedical Exemptions to State Immunization Laws," *American Journal of Public Health* 91 (2001): 645; State of Michigan, Department of Community Health, Lansing, "Immunization Waiver Form," DCH-0716, rev. March 2011.

6. National Conference of State Legislatures, "School Immunization Exemption State Laws," www.ncsl.org/issuesresearch/health/schoolimmunizationexemptionlaws /tabid/14376/default.aspx (accessed June 2, 2010); Linda E. LeFever, "Religious Exemptions from School Immunization: A Sincere Belief or a Legal Loophole?" *Pennsylvania State University Law Review* 110 (2005–6): 1047–67; Joseph W. Thompson, Shirley Tyson, Paula Card-Higginson, Richard F. Jacobs, J. Gary Wheeler, Pippa Simpson, James Bost, Kevin Ryan, and Daniel Salmon, "Impact of Addition of Philosophical Exemptions on Childhood Immunization Rates," *American Journal of Preventative Medicine* 32 (2007): 194–201; Alexandra M. Stewart, "Challenging Personal Belief Immunization Exemptions: Considering Legal Responses," *Michigan Law Review* 107 (2009): 105–9; Centers for Disease Control and Prevention, "Press Release: Many Unvaccinated Because of Philosophical Beliefs," August 21, 2008, www.cdc.gov /media/pressrel/2008/r080821.thm (accessed June 25, 2009); Saad B. Omer, William K. Y. Pan, Neal A. Halsey, Shannon Stokely, Lawrence H. Moulton, Ann Marie Navar, Mathew Pierce, and Daniel Salmon, "Nonmedical Exemptions to School Immunization Requirements: Secular Trends and Association of State Policies with Pertussis

Incidence," *Journal of the American Medical Association* 296 (2006): 1757–63; "Foolish Vaccine Exemptions," *New York Times,* October 12, 2006; Rota et al., "Processes for Obtaining Nonmedical Exemptions," 645–48.

7. Centers for Disease Control and Prevention, "Update: Vaccine Side Effects, Adverse Reactions, Contraindications, and Precautions Recommendations of the Advisory Committee on Immunization Practices (ACIP)," www.cdc.gov/mmwr/preview /mmwrhtml/00046738.htm (accessed June 2, 2010); Advisory Committee for Immunization Practices, "Diphtheria, Tetanus, and Pertussis: Recommendations for Vaccine Use and Other Preventive Measures," *Morbidity and Mortality Weekly Report* 40 (August 8, 1991).

8. Centers for Disease Control and Prevention, "CDC Rotavirus," www.cdc.gov/ rotavirus/ (accessed December 17, 2008); "Hopes and Fears for Rotavirus Vaccines," *Lancet* 365 (January 15, 2005): 190.

9. Julie Bines, "Intussusception and Rotavirus Vaccines," *Vaccine* 25 (2006): 3772–76; "Panel Favors New Vaccine for Diarrhea in Children," *New York Times,* December 13, 1997; "F.D.A. Approves Vaccine for Childhood Diarrhea," *New York Times,* September 1, 1998; Irene Pérez-Schael, María J. Guntiñas, Mireya Pérez, Vito Pagone, Ana M. Rojas, Rosabel Gonzálas, Walter Cunto, Yasutaka Hoshino, and Albert Kapikian, "Efficacy of the Rhesus Rotavirus-Based Quadrivalent Vaccine in Infants and Young Children in Venezuela," *New England Journal of Medicine* 377 (October 23, 1997): 1181–87.

10. Margaret B. Rennels, "The Rotavirus Vaccine Story: A Clinical Investigator's View," *Pediatrics* 106 (2000): 123–25; Centers for Disease Control and Prevention, "Withdrawal of Rotavirus Vaccine Recommendation," *Morbidity and Mortality Weekly Report* 48 (November 5, 1999): 1007–8; Trudy V. Murphy, Paul Gargiullo, Mehran S. Massoudi, David B. Nelson, Aisha Jumaan, Catherine Okoro, Lynn Zanardi, Sabeena Setia, Elizabeth Fair, Charles LeBaron, Melinda Wharton, and John Livengood, "Intussusception among Infants Given an Oral Rotavirus Vaccine," *New England Journal of Medicine* 344 (February 22, 2001): 564–72; "Hopes and Fears for Rotavirus Vaccines," 190; Brian R. Murphy, David M. Morens, Lone Simonsen, Robert M. Chanock, John R. La Montagne, and Albert Z. Kapikian, "Reappraisal of the Association of Intussusception with the Licensed Life Rotavirus Vaccine Challenges Initial Conclusions," *Journal of Infectious Diseases* 187 (2003): 1301–8; Lawrence K. Altman, "U.S. in a Push to Bar Vaccine Given to Infants," *New York Times,* July 16, 1999; Lawrence K. Altman, "Vaccine for Infant Diarrhea Is Withdrawn as Health Risk," *New York Times,* October 16, 1999; Lawrence K. Altman, "In Turnabout, Federal Panel Votes Against a Vaccine," *New York Times,* October 23, 1999; Food and Drug Administration, "Merck & Company, Inc., RotaTeq: Rotavirus Vaccine, Life, Oral, Pentavalent," www.fda.gov/CbER/label/rotamero21207LB1.pdf (accessed December 18, 2008); Lawrence Altman, "Promise Found in Alternative to Vaccine Barred for Babies," *New York Times,* July 23, 1999.

11. Neil Peart, "Freewill," *Permanent Waves* (1980).

CHAPTER 1: Risk and Reward

1. Centers for Disease Control and Prevention, "Vaccines: ACIP/Charter," http:// cdc.gov/vaccines/recs/ACIP/charter.htm (accessed July 20, 2010).

2. Paul Offit, Jessica Quarles, Michael A. Gerber, Charles J. Hackett, Edgar K. Marcuse, Tobias Kollman, Bruce G. Gellin, and Sarah Landry, "Addressing Parents' Concerns: Do Multiple Vaccines Overwhelm or Weaken the Infant's Immune System?" *Pediatrics* 109 (2002): 124. My state, Michigan, mandates five doses of DPT vaccine, four doses of *Haemophilus influenzae* type b vaccine, four doses of polio vaccine, two doses of MMR vaccine, three doses of hepatitis B vaccine, four doses of pneumococcal conjugate vaccine, and one dose of varicella vaccine by the time children are six years old. The State of Michigan, "Required Immunizations for Michigan Childcare Preschool Attendance," www.mi.gov/documents/PreSchoolRules_170325_7.pdf (accessed, June 24, 2009). In addition, the CDC also recommends three doses of rotavirus vaccine, yearly doses of influenza vaccine, two doses of hepatitis A vaccine, and one dose of meningococcal vaccine. Centers for Disease Control and Prevention, "Vaccines: Recs/Schedules/Child Schedule main page," www.cdc.gov/vaccines/recs/schedules/child-schedule.htm (accessed June 24, 2009); "Vaccinations of Toddlers Set a Record," *New York Times,* September 5, 2008; Centers for Disease Control and Prevention, "Press Briefing Transcripts: CDC Announces Vaccine Coverage Rates for Children Aged 19–35 Months," September 5, 2008, www.cdc.gov/media/transcripts/2008/t080905.htm (accessed September 17, 2008); Miranda Hitti, "Childhood Vaccination Rates High," WebMD Health News, http://children.webmd.com/vaccines/news/20080904/childhood-vaccination-rates-high (accessed June 23, 2009); Centers for Disease Control and Prevention, "Estimated Vaccination Coverage with Individual Vaccines and Selected Vaccination Series Among Children 19–35 Months of Age by State and Local Area, U.S. National Immunization Survey, Q3/2006-A2/2007," available at "Vaccines: Stats-Surv/NIS/Table Data for 2007," www.cdc.gov/vaccines/stats-surv/nis/data/tables_2007.htm (accessed December 18, 2008).

3. Szabo, "Refusing Kid's Vaccine More Common Among Parents"; Donald G. McNeil Jr., "When Parents Say No to Child Vaccinations," *New York Times,* November 30, 2002; "CDC Wants to Know Why Ashland Kids Are Not Vaccinated," www.kcby.com.news/local/36879409.html (accessed June 26, 2009); Derek Kravitz, "Measles on Rise as Parents Question Vaccine," *Washington Post,* August 28, 2008; Gardiner Harris, "Measles Cases Grow in Number, and Officials Blame Parents' Fear of Autism," *New York Times,* August 22, 2008; Rob Stein, "CDC Cites Largest U.S. Resurgence of Measles Since 2001," *Washington Post,* May 2, 2008; Denise Grady, "Measles in U.S. at Highest Level Since 2001," *New York Times,* May 2, 2008; Thomas May and Ross D. Silverman, "Clustering of Exemptions as a Collective Action Threat to Herd Immunity," *Vaccine* 21 (2003): 1050.

4. Committee on Government Reform, U.S. House of Representatives, "Conflict of Interest in Vaccine Policy Making, Majority Staff Report, June 15, 2000"; Randall Neustaedter, *The Vaccine Guide: Risks and Benefits for Children and Adults,* rev. ed. (Berkeley: North Atlantic Books, 2002), 24; M. Carolina Danovaro-Holliday, Allison L. Wood, and Charles W. LeBaron, "Rotavirus Vaccine and the News Media," *Journal of the American Medical Association* 287 (2002): 1455–62.

5. Vaccine Education Center at the Children's Hospital of Philadelphia, "Welcome to the Vaccine Education Center," www.chop.edu/consumer/jsp/microsite/microsite.jsp?id=75918 (accessed December 19, 2008); Centers for Disease Control and Prevention, "Update: Vaccine Side Effects, Adverse Reactions, Contraindications,

and Precautions," *Morbidity and Mortality Weekly Report* 45, September 6, 1996, 1–35.

6. Centers for Disease Control and Prevention, "CDC—Information for Parents—Vaccine Safety," www.cdc.gov/vaccinesafety/basic/parents.htm (accessed December 19, 2008); Centers for Disease Control and Prevention, "Vaccines: Vac-Gen/Side Effects," www.cdc.gov/vaccines/vac-gen/side-effects.htm (accessed December 19, 2008); The Vaccine Education Center at the Children's Hospital of Philadelphia, "Frequently Asked Questions about Vaccines," www.chop.edu/consumer/jsp/division /generic.jsp?id=75743#Are_vaccines_safe (accessed December 18, 2008); Iain Laing, "Vaccine Horror—When that 'One in a Million' is Your Child," www.rense.com/ufo6 /1inmil.htm (accessed August 23, 2010).

7. Bruce G. Gellin, Edward W. Maibach, and Edgar K. Marcuse, "Do Parents Understand Immunizations? A National Telephone Survey," *Pediatrics* 106 (2000): 1097–1102; Rick Blizzard, Glen Nowak, and Alan Janssen, "Vaccination Frequency, Side Effects Worry Parents" (June 22, 2008), www.gallup.com/poll/12097/Vaccina tion-Frequency-Side-Effects-Worry-Parents.aspx (accessed December 18, 2008).

8. Centers for Disease Control and Prevention, "Vaccines: VPD-VAC/Varicella /General Vaccine FAQs," www.cdc.gov/vaccines/vpd-vac/varicella/vac-faqs-gen.htm (accessed December 18, 2008); American Academy of Family Physicians, "Chicken-pox Vaccine—familydoctor.org," http://familydoctor.org/online/famdocen/home /healthy/vaccines/193.html (accessed December 18, 2008); American Academic of Pediatrics, "Varicella/Chickenpox," www.aap.org/immunization/illnesses/varicella /chickenpox.html (accessed August 21, 2010).

9. For an excellent discussion of the apparent American compulsion to adopt technological solutions in hopes of remedying vexing social problems, see Daniel Sarewitz, *Frontiers of Illusion: Science, Technology, and the Politics of Progress* (Phila-delphia: Temple University Press, 1996). In particular, the eighth chapter of Sare-witz's book, "Science as Surrogate for Social Action," nicely explores the way in which Americans seek techno-fixes in lieu of resolving the issues that are at the root of so-cial or political problems. For discussions of technologies that allow us to avoid deal-ing with workplace/family tensions, see Kate Boyer and Maia Boswell-Penc, "Breast Pumps: A Feminist Technology or (Yet) More Work for Mother?" in *Feminist Tech-nology* (Champaign: University of Illinois Press, 2010): 119–35.

10. Stephen R. Preblud, "Varicella: Complications and Costs," *Pediatrics* 78 (1986): 731; Sandra S. Chaves, Paul Gargiullo, John X. Zhang, Rachel Civen, Daly Guris, Laurene Mascola, and Jane F. Seward, "Loss of Vaccine-Induced Immunity to Varicella over Time," *New England Journal of Medicine* 356 (2007): 1121; "Chickenpox Vaccine Loses Effectiveness in Study," *New York Times,* March 15, 2007; "Notice to Readers: Licensure of a Combined Live Attenuated Measles, Mumps, Rubella, and Varicella Vaccine," *Morbidity and Mortality Weekly Report* 54 (2005): 1212–14.

11. Liz Austin Peterson, "Texas Gov. Orders Anti-Cancer Vaccine," *Washington Post,* February 3, 2007; Liz Austin Peterson, "Governor's Office Says Timing Is Coin-cidence, No Conspiracy Existed," *Austin Statesmen,* February 22, 2007; Associated Press, "Rick Perry's Ties with Merck Run Deep," KBTX.com, www.kbtx.com/home /headlines/5546651.html (accessed June 10, 2010).

12. Stephanie Saul and Andrew Pollack, "Furor on Rush to Require Cervical Can-cer Vaccine," *New York Times,* February 17, 2007; Andrew Pollack and Stephanie

Saul, "Merck to Halt Lobbying for Vaccine for Girls," *New York Times,* February 21, 2007; Merck & Company, Inc., "GARDASIL (Human Papillomavirus Quadrivalent [Types 5, 11, 16, and 18] Vaccine), Recombinant," www.gardasil.com (accessed December 18, 2008); Kristen Fyfe, "ABC Wakes Up, Reports Gardasil Dangers," www .cultureandmediainstitute.org/articles/2008/20080821120743.aspx (accessed December 18, 2008). See also Jessica Nickrand, "The State of Gardasil: The Political Implications of the HPV Vaccine," *The Medical Humanities Report* 29 (2008).

13. Marc-André Gagnon and Joel Lexchin, "The Cost of Pushing Pills: A New Estimate of Pharmaceutical Promotion Expenditures in the United States," *PLoS Med* 5 (2008); "Big Pharma Spends More on Advertising Than Research and Development, Study Finds," *Science Daily*, January 7, 2008, www.sciencedaily.com/re leases/2008/01/080105140107.htm (accessed June 2, 2010). A similar critique of pharmaceutical companies' expansive marketing efforts and limited expenditures on research and development is offered by Marcia Angell, the former editor of the *New England Journal of Medicine*. Angell "contends that the industry has become a marketing machine that produces few innovative drugs and is dependent on monopoly rights and public-sponsored research," and she "disputes the industry's reputation as an 'engine of innovation,' arguing that the top U.S. drug makers spend 2.5 times as much on marketing and administration as they do on research." "The Truth about Drug Companies," *Mother Jones,* September 7, 2004, http://motherjones.com/poli tics/2004/09/truth-about-drug-companies (accessed June 2, 2010); Marcia Angell, *The Truth About Drug Companies: How They Deceive Us and What to Do About It* (New York: Random House, 2005).

14. Gary L. Freed, Sarah J. Clark, Amy T. Butchart, Diane C. Singer, and Matthew M. Davis, "Parental Vaccine Concerns in 2009," *Pediatrics* 125 (2010): 654–59. Of the 2521 surveys sent to parents of children who were younger than seventeen years old, researchers obtained responses from 62 percent. Of these, 11.5 percent of the parents said that they had refused one or more of the mandated or recommended vaccines for their children. The HPV vaccine was the most commonly refused vaccine (56.4 percent), followed by varicella (32.3 percent), meningococcal conjugate (31.8 percent), and MMR (17.7 percent).

15. "Parents Claim Religion to Avoid Vaccines for Kids," *MSNBC,* October 17, 2007, www.msnbc.msn.com/id/21347434/ (accessed July 8, 2009). Among Christian Scientists, there is no prohibition against vaccination, but the church does say, "Generally, a Christian Scientist's first choice is to rely on prayer for healing, and in most cases this means that a medical remedy is unnecessary." The church expects its members to "gladly abide by city and state laws or mandates regarding quarantines, vaccinations, and the like," but also lobbies for exemptions to health laws. "Questions: Christian Science FAQs," http://christianscience.com/questions/questions -christian-science-faq/ (accessed June 21, 2010). Among the Amish, there is no direct prohibition against vaccination; however, their general practice of separation from the modern world leads to low levels of coverage for routine childhood vaccinations. Carolyn E. Adams and Michael Leverland, "The Effects of Religious Beliefs on the Health Care Practices of the Amish," *Nurse Practitioner* 11: 58–67. Among Jehovah's Witnesses, vaccination was prohibited in the 1920s, but became acceptable in the 1950s. *The Watchtower,* December 15, 1952, and "Questions from Readers," *The Watchtower,* September 15, 1958.

16. Jennifer Steinhauer, "Public Health Risk Seen as Parents Reject Vaccines," *New York Times,* March 21, 2008; Allison M. Kenney, Cedric J. Brown, and Deborah A. Gust, "Vaccine Beliefs of Parents Who Oppose Compulsory Vaccination," *Public Health Reports* 120 (2005): 256; Gellin, Maibach, and Marcuse, "Do Parents Understand Immunizations?"

17. Pontifical Academy for Life, "Moral Reflections on Vaccines Prepared from Cells Derived from Aborted Human Fetuses," *National Catholic Bioethics Quarterly* 6 (2006): 541–37. In the most recent poll on the subject, researchers found that only 11 percent of survey parents agreed with the statement "My child(ren) does (do) not need vaccines for diseases that are not common anymore"; Freed et al., "Parental Vaccine Concerns in 2009," 656.

18. Wendell Jones, "Readers' Comments, March 21, 2008, 8:43 a.m.," *New York Times* website, "Public Health Risk Seen as Parents Reject Vaccines—Readers' Comments—NYTimes.com," http://community.nytimes.com/article/comments/2008/03/21/us/21vaccine.html?permid=61#comment61 (accessed December 22, 2008); Robert W. Sears, *The Vaccine Book: Making the Right Choice for Your Child* (New York: Little, Brown and Company, 2007), 221.

19. For example, see Thomas Harding and Linus Gregoriadis, "Fears Grow of Epidemic as Parents Shun MMR Vaccine," *Telegraph,* January 5, 2002; Nic Fleming, "MMR Confusion 'Could Lead to Deaths,'" *Telegraph,* June 27, 2006; "Op-Ed: The Measles Vaccine Follies," *New York Times,* August 9, 2006; Shaoni Bhattacharya and Andy Coghlan, "MMR Fears Lead to Looming Measles Epidemic," Newscientist .com, www.newscientist.com/article.ns?id=dn4036&print=true (accessed June 9, 2008); BBC News, "MMR Vaccine Uptake Rise 'Stalls,'" http://news.bbc.co.uk/go/pr/fr/-/2/hi/health/7633115.stm (accessed September 25, 2008); Hitti, "Childhood Vaccination Rates High"; Donald G. McNeil Jr., "Sharp Drop Seen in Deaths from Ills Fought by Vaccine," *New York Times,* November 14, 2007; "Fears Rise over Measles Outbreak," BBC News, October 29, 2008, http://newsvote.bbc.co.uk/go/pr/fe/-/2/hi/uk_news/england/manchester/7697269.stm (accessed October 29, 2008); Kravitz, "Measles on Rise as Parents Question Vaccine"; McNeil, "When Parents Say No to Child Vaccines"; Grady, "Measles in U.S. at Highest Level Since 2001"; Stein, "CDC Cites Largest U.S. Resurgence of Measles Since 2001"; Harris, "Measles Cases Grow in Number, and Official Blame Parents' Fear of Autism."

20. "CDC Releases 1918 Influenza Pandemic Storybook," news-medical.net, www .news-medical.net/news/2008/08/24/40856.aspx (accessed June 9, 2010); Centers for Disease Control and Prevention, "CDC PanFlu Storybook—Home Page," www.cdc .gov/about/panflu/ (accessed June 9, 2010). I owe special thanks to Prof. Catherine Belling of Northwestern University for informing me of the CDC's Storybook project.

21. Gellin et al., "Do Parents Understand Immunizations?" 1098–99.

22. Chaïm Perelman and Lucie Olbrechts-Tyteca, *The New Rhetoric: A Treatise on Argumentation,* trans. John Wilkinson and Purcell Weaver (Notre Dame: University of Notre Dame Press, 1969), 74–75.

23. Perelman and Olbrechts-Tyteca, *The New Rhetoric,* 77–80.

24. An excellent discussion of how professions use quantification to manufacture objectivity and create normative standards can be found in Theodore M. Porter,

Trust in Numbers: The Pursuit of Objectivity in Science and Public Life (Princeton, NJ: Princeton University Press, 1995).

25. Edmund Massey, "A Sermon Against the Dangerous and Sinful Practice of Inoculation, Preach'd at St. Andrew's Holborn on Sunday, July the 8th, 1722 (London: William Meadows, 1722).

26. Michael Berube refers to this group of Americans as "Krups People." They are people "in that class/taste faction in which people own good books, drink strong coffee brewed in pricey German coffeemakers, rent foreign films . . . and paint their walls distinctive and vibrant colors." Michael Berube, "Leftwing Media Day!" www .michaelberube.com/index.php/weblog/2006/04/P12/ (accessed July 20, 2010).

27. Philip J. Smith, Susan Y. Chu, and Lawrence E. Barker, "Children Who Have Received No Vaccines: Who Are They and Where Do They Live?" *Pediatrics* 114 (2004): 188; Centers for Disease Control and Prevention, "Statistics and Surveillance: 2008 Table Data, Coverage Levels by Milestone Ages, 24 Months by State and Local Area," www2a.cdc.gov/nip/coverage/nis/nis_iap2.asp?fmt=v&rpt=tab09_24mo_iap &qtr=Q1/2008-Q4/2008 (accessed June 9, 2010).

28. Freed et al., "Parental Vaccine Concerns in 2009," 657; MSNBC, "See Your State's Vaccination Exemption Rates—Kids and Parenting—MSNBC.com," www .msnbc.msn.com/id/26337586 (accessed June 10, 2010).

29. Sam S. Kim, Jemima A. Frimpong, Patrick A. Rivers, and Jennie J. Kronenfeld, "Effects of Maternal and Provider Characteristics on Up-to-Date Immunization Status of Children Aged 19 to 35 Months," *American Journal of Public Health* 97 (2007): 259–66; Nicholas Bakalar, "Vital Signs: Immunizations; More Education May Not Mean More Vaccination," *New York Times*, January 16, 2007; Freed et al., "Parental Vaccine Concerns in 2009," 656; Deborah A. Gust, Natalie Darling, Allison Kennedy, and Ben Schwartz, "Parents with Doubts about Vaccines: Which Vaccines and Reasons Why," *Pediatrics* 122 (2008): 720, 722–23; Andrea L. Benin, Daryl J. Wisler-Scher, Eve Colson, Eugene D. Shapiro, and Eric S. Holmboe, "Qualitative Analysis of Mother's Decision-Making about Vaccines for Infants: The Importance of Trust," *Pediatrics* 117 (2006): 1532–41; Deborah Gust, Allison Kennedy, Irene Shui, Philip Smith, Glen Nowak, and Larry K. Pickering, "Parent Attitudes toward Immunizations and Healthcare Providers," *American Journal of Preventative Medicine* 29 (2005): 105–12; Gellin, Maibach, and Marcuse, "Do Parents Understand Immunizations?"

30. Gellin, Maibach, and Marcuse, "Do Parents Understand Immunizations?"; Norman A. Constantine and Petra Jerman, "Acceptance of Human Papillomavirus Vaccination among Californian Parents of Daughters: A Representative Statewide Analysis," *Journal of Adolescent Health* 40 (2007): 108–15; Norman Begg, Mary Ramsay, Joanne White, and Zoltan Bozosky, "Medicine and the Media," *British Medical Journal* 316 (1998): 561.

31. Philip J. Smith, Susan Y. Chu, and Lawrence E. Barker, "Children Who Have Received No Vaccines: Who Are They and Where Do They Live?," 187–95.

32. Steinhauer, "Public Health Risk Seen as Parents Reject Vaccines." "Readers' Comments: Public Health Risk Seen as Parents Reject Vaccines," *New York Times*, http://community.nytimes.com/comments/www.nytimes.com/2008/03/21/us/21vac cine.html (accessed August 21, 2010).

CHAPTER 2: Sources of Doubt

1. Viera Scheibner, *Vaccination: 100 Years of Orthodox Research Shows that Vaccines Represent a Medical Assault on the Immune System* (Santa Fe: New Atlantean Press, 1992), 49; David C. Classen and John Barthelow Classen, "The Timing of Pediatric Immunization and the Risk of Insulin-Dependent Diabetes Mettitus," *Infectious Diseases in Clinical Practice* 6 (1997): 449–54; "Revising Miss America's Story," *New York Times*, September 26, 1994; Gary L. Freed, Samuel L. Katz, and Sarah J. Clark, "Safety of Vaccinations: Miss America, the Media, and Public Health," *Journal of the American Medical Association* 276 (1996): 1869–1918. For example, see Donald G. McNeil Jr., "Health Officials Fear New Spread of Polio," *New York Times*, February 10, 2005; Celia W. Dugger and Donald G. McNeil Jr., "Rumor Fear and Fatigue Hinder Final Push to End Polio," *New York Times*, March 20, 2006; Cecelia Chen, "Rebellion Against the Polio Vaccine in Nigeria: Implications for Humanitarian Policy," *African Health Sciences* 4 (2004): 205–7. The claim of a possible link between the polio vaccine and HIV/AIDS originated with Tom Curtis, "The Origin of AIDS," *Rolling Stone* 626, March 19, 1992, 54–59, 61, 106, 108, and has been significantly elaborated upon by Edward Hooper, *The River: A Journey Back to the Source of HIV and AIDS* (Boston: Little & Brown, 1999). The new and expanded edition of James Jones, *Bad Blood: The Tuskegee Syphilis Experiment* (New York: Free Press, 1993) includes a concluding chapter on AIDS and African Americans' anxieties about AIDS and genocide. Edward W. Campion, "Suspicions about the Safety of Vaccines," New England Journal of Medicine 347, no.19 (2002): 1474–75; Steven Lee Myers, "U.S. Armed Forces to Be Vaccinated Against Anthrax," *New York Times*, December 16, 1997; B. Asa, Y. Cao, and R. F. Garry, "Antibodies to Squalene in Gulf War Syndrome," *Experimental and Molecular Pathology* 68 (2000): 55–64. The most complete analysis of Gulf War Syndrome concluded that the anthrax vaccine that was given to approximately 150,000 Gulf War combatants probably was not the cause of their ailments, but also asserted that it could not be definitively ruled out as a potential cause or contributing cause. Research Advisory Committee on Gulf War Veterans' Illnesses, *Gulf War Illness and the Health of Gulf War Veterans: Scientific Findings and Recommendations* (Washington, DC: U.S. Government Printing Office, 2008), 8; Holcomb B. Noble, "3 Suits Say Lyme Vaccine Caused Severe Arthritis," *New York Times*, January 19, 2009. In 1998 GlaxoSmithKline released Lymerix, a vaccine against Lyme disease. Within a few years, hundreds of people who had received the vaccine reported that they had developed serious autoimmune side effects, especially arthritis, and several class action lawsuits were filed alleging that the vaccine had caused health problems. Both the FDA and the CDC concluded that there was no connection between the vaccine and autoimmune disorders. Nonetheless, sales of Lymerix fell significantly and the vaccine was pulled from the U.S. market in 2002. "Sole Lyme Vaccine is Pulled Off Market," *New York Times*, February 28, 2002; "When a Vaccine Is Safe," *Nature* 439 (2006): 509; L. E. Nigrovic and K. M. Thompson, "The Lyme Vaccine: A Cautionary Tale," *Epidemiology and Infection* 135 (2007): 1–8; Christian Confavreux, Samy Suissa, Patricia Saddier, Valerie Bourdes, and Sandra Vukusic, "Vaccinations and the Risk of Relapse in Multiple Sclerosis," *New England Journal of Medicine* 344 (2001): 319–26; David Kirby, "Vaccine Court: Hepatitis B Shot Caused MS," *Age of Autism: Daily Web Newspaper of the Autism Epidemic*, February 3, 2009,

www.ageofautism.com/2009/02/vaccine-court-hepatitis-b-shot-causes-ms.html (accessed June 23, 2009).

2. Neil Z. Miller, *Vaccines: Are They Really Safe and Effective?* (Santa Fe: New Atlantean Press, 2008); Neil Z. Miller and Russell Blaylock, *Vaccine Safety Manual for Concerned Families and Health Practitioners* (Santa Fe: New Atlantean Press, 2010); Neil Z. Miller, *Immunization Theory vs. Reality* (Santa Fe: New Atlantean Press, 1995); Randall Neustaedter, *The Vaccine Guide: Risks and Benefits for Children and Adults*, rev. ed. (Berkeley: North Atlantic Books, 2002); Neustaedter, *The Immunization Decision* (Berkeley: North Atlantic Books, 1990); Neustaedter, *Flu: Alternative Treatments and Prevention* (Berkeley: North Atlantic Books, 2004); Robert S. Mendelsohn, *How to Raise a Healthy Child in Spite of Your Doctor* (New York: Ballantine Books, 1987); Mendelsohn, *Confessions of a Medical Heretic* (Chicago: Contemporary Books, 1979).

3. An example of the use of the term *biomedical approach* can be found in the work of Robert Sears, of the widely read Dr. Sears family and coauthor of the Sears Parenting Library. He wrote, "The biomedical approach is a very different world; a world that your regular physician may scoff at; a world not approved by the FDA. But it's a world that I've been involved with since 2000 and one that I will continue to be part of until it merges with mainstream medicine. Then I won't have to refer to it as *alternative* anymore." Robert W. Sears, *The Autism Book: What Every Parent Needs to Know about Early Detection, Treatment, Recovery, and Prevention* (New York: Little, Brown and Co., 2010), 78.

4. Tim Horder, "Roger Sperry and Integrative Action in the Nervous System," in *Rebels, Mavericks, and Heretics in Biology*, ed. Oren Harman and Michael Dietrich (New Haven: Yale University Press, 2008), 174.

5. Karl Popper, *The Logic of Scientific Discovery* (New York: Basic Books, 1959). While in theory scientific claims are under constant challenge, in practice journals are much more inclined to publish original articles and reluctant to publish refutations. For a nice discussion of this, see Carl Zimmer, "It's Science, But Not Necessarily Right," *New York Times*, June 25, 2011.

6. The historian of science John P. Jackson Jr., described how falsificationism requires a post hoc assessment in John P. Jackson Jr., "Fact, Values, and Policies: A Comment on Howard H. Kendler (2002)," *History of Psychology* 6 (2003): 200.

7. David M. Eisenberg, Roger B. Davis, Susan L. Ettner, Scott Appel, Sonja Wilkey, Maria Van Rompay, and Ronald C. Kessler, "Trends in Alternative Medicine Use in the United States 1990–1997: Results of a Follow-Up National Survey," *Journal of the American Medical Association* 280 (1998): 1569–75.

8. The tension between professionalism and egalitarianism is explored in Samuel Haber, "The Professions," in *Encyclopedia of American Social History*, ed. Mary Kupiec Cayton, Elliott J. Gorn, and Peter W. Williams (New York: Scribners, 1993): II, 1573–88. Samuel Haber, *The Quest for Authority and Honor in the American Professions, 1750–1900* (Chicago: University of Chicago Press, 1991); private correspondence between the author and John P. Jackson Jr., July 19, 2010.

9. Jason W. Busse, Lon Morgan, and James B. Campbell, "Chiropractic Anti-vaccination Arguments," *Journal of Manipulative and Physiological Therapies* 28 (2005): 368.

10. J. B. Campbell, J. W. Busse, and H. S. Injyean, "Chiropractors and Vaccinations: A Historical Perspective," *Pediatrics* 105, no. 4 (2000): 1. The authors cite

V. Gielow, *Old Dad Chiro* (Davenport, IA: Bawden Brothers Press, 1981). Bobby Westbrooks, "The Troubled Legacy of Harvey Lillard: The Black Experience in Chiropractic," *Chiropractic History* 2 (1982): 47–53; Steven C. Martin, "Chiropractic and the Social Context of Medical Technology, 1895–1925," *Technology and Culture* 34 (1993): 811.

11. Martin, "Chiropractic and the Social Context of Medical Technology," 812. Martin cites Daniel David Palmer, *The Chiropractors Adjuster: Textbook of the Science, Art and Philosophy of Chiropractic for Students and Practitioners* (Portland: Portland Printing House, 1910); Barlett Joshua Palmer, *The Science of Chiropractic*, 3rd ed. (Davenport, IA: Palmer School of Chiropractic Publisher, 1917); Martin, "Chiropractic and the Social Context of Medical Technology," 813. For more detailed discussions of the religious elements in chiropractic, see Catherine Albanese, *Nature Religion in America: From the Algonkian Indians to the New Age* (Chicago: University of Chicago Press, 1990); Robert Fuller, *Alternative Medicine and American Religious Life* (New York: Oxford University Press, 1989); James Whorton, *Crusaders for Fitness: The History of American Health Reformers* (Princeton, NJ: Princeton University Press, 1982).

12. M. L. Kimbrough, "Jailed Chiropractors: Those Who Blazed the Trail," *Chiropractic History* 18 (1998): 79–100.

13. Dan Cherkin, "AMA Policy on Chiropractic," *American Journal of Public Health* 79 (1989): 1569–70; *Wilk v. American Medical Association*, 895 F.2d 352 (7th Cir., 1990).

14. H. Ni, C. Simile, and A. M. Hardy, "Utilization of Complementary and Alternative Medicine by United States Adults," *Medical Care* 40 (2002): 353–58; A. P. Rafferty, H. B. McGee, C. E. Miller, and M. Reyes, "Prevalence of Complementary and Alternative Medicine Use: State-Specific Estimates from the 2001 Behavioral Risk Factor Surveillance System," *American Journal of Public Health* 92 (2002): 1598–1600.

15. Bartlett Joshua Palmer, *The Philosophy Chiropractic* (Davenport, IA: Palmer School of Chiropractic Publishing, 1909); Campbell, Busee, and Injeyan, "Chiropractors and Vaccination," 2. Palmer, *The Chiropractor's Adjustor*, 854; Jason W. Busse, Lon Morgan, and James B. Campbell, "Chiropractic Anti-vaccination Arguments," *Journal of Manipulative and Physiological Therapeutics* 28 (2005): 371.

16. Campbell, Busse, and Injeyan, "Chiropractors and Vaccination," 3; American Chiropractic Association, "ACA—Policies," www.acatoday.org/level2_css.cfm?T1ID=10&T2ID=117#106 (accessed June 22, 2010).

17. "Kids First," *The Hamilton Spectator*, March 14, 1998; cited in Campbell, Busse, and Injeyan, "Chiropractors and Vaccination," 4.

18. "Letter to the Editor," *Burlington Post*, May 12, 1999; cited in Busse, Morgan, Campbell, "Chiropractic Anti-vaccination Arguments," 368.

19. Campbell, Busse, Injeyan, "Chiropractors and Vaccination," 4.

20. Jason W. Busse, Abhaya V. Kulkarni, James B. Campbell, and H. Stephen Injeyan, "Attitudes Toward Vaccination: A Survey of Canadian Chiropractic Students," *Canadian Medical Association Journal* 166 (2002): 1531–34; Robert Pless and Beth Hibbs, "Chiropractic Students' Attitudes about Vaccination: A Cause for Concern?" *Canadian Medical Association Journal* 166 (2002): 1544–45.

21. Busse, Morgan, Campbell, "Chiropractic Anti-vaccination Arguments," 371.

22. Centers for Disease Control and Prevention, "Update on Acquired Immune Deficiency Syndrome (AIDS)," *Morbidity and Mortality Weekly Report* 31 (1982): 507–8; F. Barre-Sinoussi, J. C. Chermann, F. Rey, M. T. Nugeyre, S. Chamaret, J. Gruest, C. Dauguet, C. Axley-Blin, F. Vezinet-Brun, C. Rouzioux, W. Rozenbaum, and L. Montagnier, "Isolation of T-Lymphotropic Retrovirus from a Patient at Risk for Acquired Immune Deficiency Syndrome (AIDS)," *Science* 220 (1983): 868–71; R. C. Gallo, P. S. Sarin, E. P. Gelmann, M. Robert-Guroff, E. Richardson, V. S. Kalyanaraman, D. Man, G. D. Sidhu, R. E. Stahl, S. Zolla-Pazner, J. Leibowitch, and M. Popovic," *Science* 220 (1983): 865–67; J. Coffin, A. Haase, J. A. Levy, L. Montagnier, S. Oroszlan, N. Teich, H. Temin, K. Toyoshima, H. Varmus, and P. Vogt, "What To Call the AIDS Virus?" *Nature* 321 (1986): 10; Philippe Lemey, Oliver G. Pybus, Bin Wang, Nitin K. Saksena, Marco Salemi, and Anne-Mieke Vandamme, "Tracing the Origin and History of the HIV-2 Epidemic," *Proceedings of the National Academy of Science of the United States of America* 100 (2003): 6588–92.

23. Laura Lee, "Vaccines and AIDS: Interview of Dr. Eva Snead by Laura Lee," www.whale.to/vaccines/snead2.html (accessed July 1, 2010); Louis Pascal, "When Science Goes Bad: The Corruption of Science and the Origin of AIDS; A Study in Spontaneous Generation" (1991), www.uow.edu.au/~bmartin/dissent/documents/AIDS/Pascal91.html#Mfn3 (accessed July 1, 2010); Raanan Gillon, "A Startling 19,000-Word Thesis on the Origin of AIDS: Should the JME Have Published It?" *Journal of Medical Ethics* 18 (1992): 3–4.

24. Blaine F. Elswood and R. B. Stricker, "Letter to the Editor: Polio Vaccines and the Origin of AIDS," *Research in Virology* 144 (1993): 175–77. See also Blaine F. Elswood and R. B. Stricker, "Polio Vaccines and the Origins of AIDS," *Medical Hypotheses* 42 (1994): 347–54; Tom Curtis, "The Origin of AIDS," *Rolling Stone* 626, March 19, 1992, 54–108; Brad Tyler, "The Man Who Knew Too Soon," *Houston Press*, January 20, 2000.

25. Michael Le Page, "Does SV40 Contamination Matter?" *New Scientist* (July 10, 2004); "Origin of AIDS: Update," *Rolling Stone*, December 9, 1993, 39; Martin, "Sticking a Needle into Science: The Case of Polio Vaccines and the Origin of AIDS," *Social Studies of Science* 26 (1996): 252.

26. Jon Cohen, "Debate on AIDS Origin: *Rolling Stone* Weighs In," *Science* 255 (1992): 1505; C. Basilico, C. Buck, R. Desrosiers, D. Ho, R. Lilly, and E. Wimmer, "Report from the AIDS/Poliovirus Advisory Committee," unpublished, cited in Martin, "Sticking a Needle into Science," 252, 271–72.

27. For reviews of *The River*, see Tony Barnett, "Review of *The River: A Journey to the Source of HIV and AIDS*," *New Statesman Review*, July 30, 2000; Robert Trivers, "Review of *The River*," *Times Higher Education Supplement*, February 17, 2000; Marlene Cimons, "Review of *The River*," *Los Angeles Times*, December 23, 1999; Carol Ann Campbell, "Virus Evolved from Clinton Prison Polio Vaccine, Author Contends," *Star-Ledger* (Newark), December 26, 1999; Jerome Groopman, "*The River*," *The New Republic*, December 27, 1999; Brian Martin, "Review of *The River*," *Science as Culture* 9 (2000): 109–13; Laurie Garrett, "New Book Charges 1950s Polio Vaccine Spread AIDS in Africa," *Newsday*, December 14, 1999; Ruaridh Nicoll, "Article Concerning *The River*," *The Scotsman*, June 24, 2000; Roy Porter, "Review of *The River*,"

London Review of Books 22, March 2000; Matt Ridley, "Was Polio Vaccine the Cause of AIDS? Review of *The River*," *Daily Telegraph*, March 1, 2000.

28. AIDSOrigins, "Edward Hooper Biography," www.aidsorigins.com/content/view/23/30/ (accessed July 8, 2010); Jon Cohen, "Forensic Epidemiology: Vaccine Theory of AIDS Disputed at Royal Society," *Science* 15 (2000): 1850–51; "H.I.V. Link to Polio Vaccine Is Discredited by New Study," *New York Times*, April 23, 2004; David M. Hillis, "AIDS: Origins of HIV," *Science* (2000): 1757–59; Karen Birmingham, "Results Make a Monkey of OPV-AIDS Theory," *Nature Medicine* 6 (2000): 1067; Jon Cohen, "AIDS Origins: Disputed AIDS Theory Dies Its Final Death," *Science* 27 (2001): 615; Henrik Poinar, Melanie Kuch, and Svante Pääbo, "Molecular Analyses of Oral Polio Vaccine Samples," *Science* 292 (2001): 743–44.

29. Walter S. Kyle, "Simian Retroviruses, Poliovaccine, and Origin of AIDS," *Lancet* 339 (1992): 600–601. In support of his claim that physicians had used monthly doses of the oral polio vaccine to treat recurrent herpes, Kyle cited C. Lincoln and R. Nordstron, "Sabin Polio Vaccine for Herpes Simplex," *Schoch Letter* 25 (1976): 65–71, and A. Tager, "Preliminary Report on the Treatment of Recurrent Herpes Simples with Poliomyelitis Vaccine," *Dermatologica* (1974): 253–55.

30. Zhores A. Medvedev, "Letter to the Editor: AIDS Virus Infection; A Soviet View of Its Origin," *Journal of the Royal Society of Medicine* 79 (1986): 494; John Seale, "Reply: AIDS Virus Infection; A Soviet View of Its Origin," *Journal of the Royal Society of Medicine* 79 (1986): 494–95. According to Seale, Zapevalov first asserted that scientists working for the Pentagon in Fort Detrick, Maryland, and at the CDC created HIV by injecting humans with animal viruses in an October 30, 1985, article entitled "Panic in the West: Or What Hides Behind the Sensationalism of AIDS," which was published in *Literaturnaya Gazeta*, which was the official weekly of the Soviet Writers' Union. Two months later the same journal published an extensive interview with Professor S. Drozdov, the Director of the Research Institute of Poliomyelitis and Encephalitis of the Academy of Medical Sciences of the USSR in which he likewise suggested that HIV was a man-made virus. Boyd E. Graves, *State Origin: The Evidence of the Laboratory Birth of Aids; A Shocking Collection of Evidence and Court Documents from* Graves vs. the President of the United States, *U.S. Supreme Court Case No. 00-9587* (Abilene, KS: National Organization for the Advancement of Humanity & Zygote Media, 2001); Juliet Lapidos, "The AIDS Conspiracy Handbook: Jeremiah Wright's Paranoia, in Context," *Slate*, www .slate.com/id/2186860 (accessed July 7, 2010); Junious Ricardo Stanton, "Boyd Graves AIDS Activist: Takes on the U.S. Government," *ChickenBones: A Journal for Literary and Artistic African-American Themes*, www.nathanielturner.com/boydgraves aidsactivist.htm (accessed July 7, 2010); Lanny Messinger, "Dr. Gary Glum, Essiac and the Antidote for AIDS," www.healthfreedom.info/Essiac percent20AIDS.htm (accessed July 10, 2010); Gary Glum, *Full Disclosure: The Truth about the AIDS Epidemic* (Los Angeles: Silent Walker Publishing, 1994); Alan Cantwell Jr., *AIDS and the Doctors of Death: An Inquiry into the Origin of the AIDS Epidemic* (Los Angeles: Aries Rising Press, 1988); Alan Cantwell Jr., *AIDS, the Mystery and the Solution* (Los Angeles: Aries Rising Press, 1988); Alan Cantwell Jr., *Queer Blook: The Secret AIDS Genocide Plot* (Los Angeles: Aries Rising Press, 1993); Neil Z. Miller, *Immunization Theory vs. Reality: Exposé on Vaccinations* (Santa Fe: New Atlantean Press, 1996, 1999), 55–62. Alan Cantwell Jr., "Rev. Jeremiah Wright Is Right about Man-Made

AIDS," Conspiracy Planet: The Alternative News and History Network, www.con
spiracyplanet.com/channel.cfm?channelid=34&contentid=5035&page=2 (accessed
July 10, 2010).

31. Darryl Fears, "Study: Many Blacks Cite AIDS Conspiracy," *Washington Post*,
January 25, 2005; Juliet Lapidos, "The AIDS Conspiracy Handbook: Jeremiah
Wright's Paranoia, in Context," *Slate*, www.slate.com/id/2186860 (accessed July 10,
2010); "Obama's Ex-Pastor Cancels Speeches," www.foxnews.com/wires/2008Mar26
/0,4670,ObamaPastor,00.html (accessed July 7, 2010). "Reverend Jeremiah Wright
Was Right about Man-Made AIDS," *Paranoia: The Conspiracy and Paranormal
Reader* 48 (2008): 34–39.

32. Walter Gibbs, "Nobel Peace Laureate Seeks to Explain Remarks about AIDS,"
New York Times, December 10, 2004; Donald G. McNeil Jr., "New Concern on Polio
among Mecca Pilgrims," *New York Times*, February 11, 2005; Donald G. McNeil Jr.,
"Muslims' New Tack on Polio: A Vaccine en Route to Mecca," *New York Times*, August 20, 2005.

33. Donald G. McNeil Jr., "Precursor to H.I.V. Was in Monkeys for Millenia,"
New York Times, September 16, 2010.

34. "Gary Null: Your Guide to Natural Living," www.garynull.com/about-gary
(accessed July 3, 2010); Gary Null, "Vaccination Nation," www.vaccinenation.net
/(accessed July 4, 2010); Gary Null, "Flu Vaccines: Are They Effective and Safe?" www
.garynull.com/storage/pdfs/SwineFluWhitePaper.pdf (accessed July 3, 2010); Richard
Gale and Gary Null, "Bracing Ourselves for More Sham Vaccine Studies: The National Institute of Allergy and Infectious Diseases Addiction to Bad Science," www
.garynull.com/storage/pdfs/ShamVaccine.pdf (accessed July 3, 2010).

35. Raanan Gillon, "A Startling 19,000-Word Thesis on the Origins of AIDS:
Should the JME Have Published It? *Journal of Medical Ethics* 29, no. 4 (August 2003):
3–4; Pascal, "When Science Goes Bad"; "Editorial: Time for a Truce?" *Nature* 407
(2000): 115; John P. Moore, "Up the River without a Paddle?: The Theory that Polio-
Vaccine Researchers Are Responsible for AIDS Is Leaky," *Nature* 401 (1999): 325–26.
Hooper responded to Moore's review in a letter for the editor of *Nature*, claiming
that Moore had made a number of factual errors in his review. The editor chose not
to publish Hooper's letter. It can be found at www.aidsorigins.com/content/view/136
/26/ (accessed July 7, 2010). David Dickson, "Tests Fail to Support Claims for Origin
of AIDS in Polio Vaccine," *Nature* 407 (2000): 117.

36. Michael Worobey, Mario L. Santiago, Brandon F. Keele, Jean-Bosco N.
Ndjango, Jeffrey B. Joy, Bernard L. Labama, Benoît D. Dhed'a, Andrew Rambaut,
Paul M. Sharp, George M. Shaw, and Beatrice H. Hahn, "Contaminated Polio Vac-
cine Theory Refuted," *Nature* (April 22, 2004): 820; "H.I.V. Link to Polio Vaccine Is
Discredited by New Study," *New York Times*, April 23, 2004.

37. Angela Hudson, "Correspondence: The Origin of AIDS," *Rolling Stone*, April
30, 1992; Gina Kolata, "Theory Tying AIDS to Polio Vaccine Is Discounted," *New
York Times*, October 23, 1992.

38. Susan P. Proctor, Roberta F. White, Timothy Heeren, Frodi Debes, Birte
Gloerfelt-Tarp, Merete Appleyard, Toben Ishoy, Bernadette Guldager, Poul Suadi-
cani, Finn Gyntelberg, and David M. Ozonoff, "Neuropsychological Functioning in
Danish Gulf War Veterans," *Journal of Pscyhopathology and Behavioral Assessment*
25 (2003): 85.

39. Anthony H. Cordesman, *Iraq and the War of Sanctions: Conventional Threats and Weapons of Mass Destruction* (Santa Barbara: Praeger, 1999), 402.

40. Barbara LaClair, "Overview of Exposures and Health Conditions Reported by Countries Who Served in the 1990–1991 Gulf War Allied Coalition," Minutes of the Meeting of the Research Advisory Committee on Gulf War Veterans' Illnesses, December 12, 2005, 73. Meetings can be found at www1.va.gov/RAC-GWVI/docs /Minutes_and_Agendas/Minutes_Dec2005_AppendixA_Presentation01.pdf (accessed July 8, 2010); *Bates v. Rumsfeld*, 271 F.Supp.2d 54 (D.D.C. 2002); *United States v. Washington*, 57 M.J. 394, 399 (C.A.A.F.2002); *Mazares v. Department of the Navy*, 302 F.3d 1382 (Fed. Cir. 2002); *Barber v. United States Army*, No. 03-1056 (10th Cir. December 18, 2003) (unpublished); *John Doe #1 v. Rumsfeld*, F.Supp.2d, 2003 WL 22994225 (D.D.C., December 22, 2003); "Pentagon to Require Some Anthrax Vaccinations," *New York Times*, October 17, 2006; "Pentagon to Resume Forced Anthrax Vaccine Program," *New York Times*, October 17, 2006.

41. Department of Veterans Affairs, "Q's and A's Regarding Birth Defects," *Gulf War Review* 12 (2003): 10; Barbara LaClair, "Overview of Exposures and Health Conditions Reported by Countries Who Served in the 1990–1991 Gulf War Allied Coalition," presentation to the Department of Veterans' Affairs Research Advisory Committee on Gulf War Veterans' Illnesses (December 12–13, 2005), Washington, DC, 70–71.

42. Janet Raloff, "Gulf War Syndrome Real, Institute of Medicine Concludes: Genetic Vulnerability May Explain Why Only Some Troops Have Been Effected," *Science News*, April 10, 2010.

43. Miller, *Immunization Theory vs. Reality*, 63–72.

44. Gary Null, *Germs, Biological Warfare, Vaccinations: What You Need to Know* (New York: Seven Stories Press, 2003), 101, 197–260.

45. Gary Matsumoto, *Vaccine A: The Covert Government Experiment That's Killing Our Soldiers and Why GI's Are Only the First Victims* (New York: Basic Books, 2004), xiii, xvi, xix.

46. Richard H. Pitcairn, "A New Look at the Two Popular Forms of Alternative Medicine, Homeopathy and Naturopathy, Have Both Had Long-Standing Vaccine Question," www.bestfrisbeedogs.com/vaccinequestion.html (accessed July 10, 2010); Laura Wallingford, "Vaccinosis: Dr. Richard Pitcairn Discusses Chronic Disease Caused by Vaccines," *Wolf Clan Magazine* (1985); "Vaccinosis," *Tiger Tribe* (1992), www.petresource.com/Articlespercent20ofpercent20Interest/vaccinosis.htm (accessed July 10, 2010); Y. Shoenfeld and A. Aron-Maor, "Vaccination and Autoimmunity—'Vaccinosis': A Dangerous Liaison?" *Journal of Autoimmunity* 14 (2000): 1–10; Janet Raloff, "Gulf War Syndrome Real, Institute of Medicine Concludes," *Science News*, April 10, 2010. The strongest example of claims about a genetic predisposition to autism that I found came from Robert Sears's 2008 *The Autism Book* in his discussion of the principal cause of autism. "We believe that the majority of children with autism are born healthy and neurologically normal but may have some genetic abnormalities that set them up for autism. During the first few years of life, a child is exposed to a variety of factors that work together to trigger autism. While these factors will be harmless to most children, taken together in a genetically susceptible child, they add up and cause a gradual (or in some cases rapid) decline into autism" (79).

47. Null, *Germs, Biological Warfare, Vaccinations*, 105–6. Null cites Julie Klotter, "Antthrax [*sic*] Vaccine," *Townsend Letter for Doctors and Patients* (January 2002): 1. Google, "william crowe bioport" (accessed July 10, 2010).

48. Abraham Maslow, *The Psychology of Science: A Reconnaissance* (Chicago: Henry Regnery Co., 1966, 1969), 15–16.

CHAPTER 3: Thimerosal and Autism

1. Hans Asperger, "Das Psychisch Abnormale Kind," *Wien Klin Wochenschr* 51 (1938): 1314–17; Leo Kanner, "Autistic Disturbances of Affective Contact," *Nervous Child* 2 (1943): 217–50.

2. Francesca Happé, Angelica Ronald, and Robert Plomin, "Time to Give Up on a Single Explanation for Autism," *Nature Neuroscience* 9 (2006): 1218–20.

3. California Department of Developmental Services, "Changes in the Population with Autism and Pervasive Developmental Disorders in California's Developmental Services System: 1987–1998; A Report to the Legislature" (Sacramento: California Health and Human Services Agency, 1999); Rick Weiss, "1 in 150 Children in U.S. Has Autism, New Survey Finds," *Washington Post*, February 9, 2007; Autism and Developmental Disabilities Monitoring Network 2006 Principal Investigators, "Prevalence of Autism Spectrum Disorder—Autism and Developmental Disabilities Monitoring Network, United States, 2006," *Morbidity and Mortality Weekly Report* 58 (December 18, 2009): 1–20; Barry Morrow and Ronald Bass, *Rain Man* (1988): "A Mysterious Upsurge in Autism," *New York Times,* October 20, 2002; "Baffling Rise in Childhood Autism: No Explanation for Sharp Increase among California Children," *CBS NEWS*, October 18, 2002; J. Madeleine Nash and Amy Bonesteel, "The Secrets of Autism," *Time*, May 6, 2002, 48; NBC, "The Marino Family's Fight Against Autism," *Today Show*, February 22, 2005; "Doug Flutie Jr. Foundation for Autism," www.doug flutiejrfoundation.org (accessed January 6, 2009); CNN, "Interview with Don and Deirdre Imus," *Larry King Live*, March 21, 2006. For discussions of the so-called autism epidemic, see Kenneth Bock and Cameron Stauth, *Healing the New Childhood Epidemics: Autism, ADHD, Asthma, and Allergies; The Groundbreaking Program for the 4-A Disorders* (New York: Ballantine Books, 2007); and David Kirby, *Evidence of Harm: Mercury in Vaccines and the Autism Epidemic; A Medical Controversy* (New York: St. Martin's Griffin, 2005). It should be noted that since the publication of *Evidence of Harm*, Kirby has revised his claim about the link between vaccines and autism by stating that the disorders he believes vaccines cause in some children are inaccurately diagnosed as autism. In a posting on *The Huffington Post* in 2007, Kirby wrote, "Maybe what these kids have is not autism, but something like, say 'Environmentally-Acquired Neuroimmune Disorder,' which we could call E.N.D. (Great slogan. 'Let's End E.N.D.')." David Kirby, "There Is No Autism Epidemic," *The Huffington Post,* www.huffingtonpost.com/david-kirby/there-is-no-autism-epidem _b_37647.html (accessed January 6, 2009).

4. S. Folstein and M. Rutter, "Infantile Autism: A Genetic Study of 21 Twin Pairs," *Journal of Child Psychology and Psychiatry and Allied Disciplines* 18 (1977): 297–321: A. Bailey, A. Le Couteur, I. Gottesman, and P. Bolton, "Autism as a Strongly Genetic Disorder: Evidence from a British Twin Study," *Psychological Medicine: A Journal of Research in Psychiatry and the Allied Sciences* 25 (1995): 63–77. For discussions of the

problematic notion of a genetic epidemic, "No Such Thing as a Genetic Epidemic," *Left Brian Right Brain*, May 15, 2008, http://leftbrainrightbrain.co.uk/2008/05/no -such-thing-as-a-genetic-epidemic/ (accessed July 14, 2010); and "But It Can't Be a Genetic Epidemic!, or Dumbasses Piling Up and a Rant (Lucy You!)," *Counter Age of Autism*, June 16, 2010, http://counteringageofautism.blogspot.com/2010/06/but-it-cant -be-genetic-epidemic-or.html (accessed July 14, 2010).

5. Alan Zarembo, "Autism Study Downplays Role of Genetics," *Los Angeles Times*, July 5, 2011; Malin Larsson, Bernard Weiss, Staffan Janson, Jan Sundell, and Carl-Gustav Bornehag, "Associations between Indoor Environmental Factors and Parental-Reported Autistic Spectrum Disorders in Children 6–8 Years of Age," *Neuro-Toxicology* 30 (2009): 822–31; Dennis K. Kinney, Daniel H. Barch, Bogdan Chayka, Siena Napoleon, and Kermin M. Munir, "Environmental Risk Factors for Autism: Do They Help Cause *De Novo* Genetic Mutations that Contribute to the Disorder?" *Medical Hypotheses* 74 (2010): 102–6; Richard Lathe, "Environmental Factors and Limbic Vulnerability in Childhood Autism," *American Journal of Biochemistry and Biotechnology* 4 (2008): 183–97; Richard Deth, Christina Muratore, Jorge Benzecry, Verna-Ann Power-Charnitsky, and Mostafa Waly, "How Environmental and Genetic Factors Combine to Cause Autism: A Redox/Methylation Hypothesis," *NeuroToxicology* 29 (2008): 190–201; Perri Klass, "Environment Poses a Knotty Challenge in Autism," *New York Times*, August 8, 2011.

6. Lorna Wing, "Editorial: Autistic Spectrum Disorders," *British Medical Journal* 312 (1996): 327–28; Eric Fombonne, "Is There an Epidemic of Autism?" *Pediatrics* 107 (2001): 411–12; Lorna Wing and David Potter, "The Epidemiology of Autistic Spectrum Disorders: Is the Prevalence Rising?" *Mental Retardation and Developmental Disabilities* 8 (2002): 151–61; Eric Fombonne, "The Prevalence of Autism," *Journal of the American Medical Association* 289 (2003): 87–89; M. Rutter, "Incidence of Autism Spectrum Disorders: Changes Over Time and Their Meaning," *Acta Paediatrica* 94 (2005): 2–15; Ashley Wazana, Michaeline Bresnahan, and Jennie Kline, "The Autism Epidemic: Fact or Artifact?" *Journal of the American Academy of Child and Adolescent Psychiatry* 46 (2007): 721–30; Arthur Allen, "The Autism Numbers: Why There's No Epidemic," *Slate*, www.slate.com/toolbar.aspx?action=print&id=2157496 (accessed January 6, 2008); Morton Ann Gernsbacher, Michelle Dawson, and H. Hill Goldsmith, "Three Reasons Not to Believe in an Autism Epidemic," *Current Directions in Psychological Science* 14 (2005): 55–58; Roy Richard Grinker, *Unstrange Minds: Remapping the World of Autism* (New York: Basic Books, 2007), 153; Edward W. Campion, "Suspicions about the Safety of Vaccines," 1474; B. Taylor, "Vaccines and the Changing Epidemiology of Autism," *Child: Care, Health and Development* 32 (2006): 511–19.

7. F. Edward Yazbak, "Autism in the United States: A Perspective," *Journal of American Physicians and Surgeons* 8 (2003): 103–7. Another example of this can be found in Mark F. Blaxill, David S. Basking, and Walter O. Spitzer, "Commentary: Blaxill, Baskin, and Spitzer on Croen et al. (2002), The Changing Prevalence of Autism in California," *Journal of Autism and Developmental Disorders* 33 (2003): 223–26. Blaxill was a member of the Board of Directors for *SafeMinds*, which is "a nonprofit organization founded to investigate and raise awareness of the risks to infants and children of exposure to mercury from medical products, including thimerosal in vaccines." www.safeminds.org/ (accessed July 7, 2009). Baskin was the cochair of

the Scientific Review Council for the Cure Autism Now Foundation, which has recently merged with Autism Speaks. A response to Blaxill's, Blaskin's, and Spitzer's commentary can be found in Lisa A. Croen and Judith Grether, "Response: A Response to Blaxill, Baskin, and Spitzer on Croen et al. (2002), 'The Changing Prevalence of Autism in California,'" *Journal of Autism and Developmental Disorders* 33 (2003): 227–29.

8. Mayo Clinic, "Autism. Causes—MayoClinic.com," www.mayoclinic.com/health/autism/DS00348/DSECTION=causes (accessed June 12, 2010); Mayo Clinic, "Autism Prevention—MayoClinic.com," www.mayoclinic.com/health/autism/DS00348/DSECTION=prevention (accessed June 12, 2010).

9. Sears, *The Autism Book: What Every Parent Needs to Know about Early Detection, Treatment, Recovery, and Prevention* (New York: Little, Brown and Company, 2010), 61, 79, 327.

10. "Parents Still Fear Autism Could Be Linked to Vaccines, Poll Shows," *Science Daily*, October 4, 2008, www.sciencedaily.com/releases/2008/10/081003122536.htm (accessed December 19, 2008); Centers for Disease Control and Prevention, "Immunization Safety and Autism," www.cdc.gov/vaccinesafety/00_pdf/VSD_Chart_of_Autism_Studies-Updated_Aug_18_09.pdf (accessed November 22, 2010).

11. U.S. Department of Health and Human Services, U.S. Food and Drug Administration, "Food and Drug Administration Modernization Act (FDAMA) of 1997," www.fda.gov/RegulatoryInformation/Legislation/FederalFoodDrugandCosmeticActFDCAct/SignificantAmendmentstotheFDCAct/FDAMA/default.htm (accessed July 12, 2010). "Food and Drug Administration Modernization Act of 1997," Public Law 105-115, 105th Congress. The request for opinions on regulation stated, "Such regulations, to the extent feasible, should not unnecessarily interfere with the availability of mercury for use in religious ceremonies." Apparently, certain Latino and Afro-Caribbean religious sects use elemental mercury in religious ceremonies. This include Sanataria, Voodoo, and Espiritismo, which wear mercury amulets, sprinkle it on the floor, or add it to a candle or oil lamp based on a belief that it is invested with magical properties and can attract luck, love, or wealth. Philip W. Davidson, Gary J. Myers, and Bernard Weiss, "Mercury Exposure and Child Development Outcomes," *Pediatrics* 113 (2004): 1023–29; Paul A. Offit, "Thimerosal and Vaccines—A Cautionary Tale," *New England Journal of Medicine* 357 (2007): 1278–79; Arthur Allen, *Vaccine: The Controversial Story of Medicine's Greatest Lifesaver* (New York: W. W. Norton & Co., 2007), 377.

12. "putchildrenfirst.com," advertisement, *USA Today* (April 6, 2006).

13. U.S. Environmental Protection Agency, "Health Effects | Mercury | US EPA," www.epa.gov/hg/effects.htm (accessed July 12, 2010); U.S. Environmental Protection Agency, "Human Exposure | Mercury | US EPA," www.epa.gov/hg/exposure.htm (accessed July 12, 2010); National Resources Defense Council, "NRDC: Mercury Contamination in Fish—Eating Tuna Safely," www.nrdc.org/health/effects/mercury/tuna.asp (accessed July 12, 2010); Ball, Ball, and Pratt, "An Assessment of Thimerosal Use in Childhood Vaccines," 1150.

14. Ball et al., "An Assessment of Thimerosal Use in Childhood Vaccines"; R. H. Bernier, "Transition Public Health Service Immunization Options," Transcript of the National Vaccine Advisory Committee Workshop on Thimerosal in Vaccines, Bethesda, Maryland (August 12, 1999); G. Stajich, G. Lopez, S. Harry and W. Saxson,

"Iatrogenic Exposure to Mercury Following Hepatitis B Vaccination in Preterm Infants," *Journal of Pediatrics* 16 (2000): 679–81.

15. Centers for Disease Control and Prevention, "Notice to Readers: Thimerosal in Vaccines; A Joint Statement of the American Academy of Pediatrics and the Public Health Service," *Morbidity and Mortality Weekly Report* 48 (1999): 563–65; Food and Drug Administration, "FDA/CBER—Thimerosal in Vaccines," www.fda.gov/cber /vaccine/thimerosal.htm (accessed December 23, 2008); Ball et al., "An Assessment of Thimerosal Use in Childhood Vaccines."

16. Thomas Burbacher, Danny D. Shen, Noelle Liberato, Kimberly S. Grant, Elsa Cernichiari, Thomas Clarkson, "Comparison of Blood and Brain Mercury Levels in Infant Monkeys Exposed to Methylmercury or Vaccines Containing Thimerosal," *Environmental Health Perspectives* 113 (2005): 1015–21.

17. World Health Organization, Global Advisory Committee on Vaccine Safety, "Statement on Thiomersal," www.who.int/vaccine_safety/topics/thiomersal/state ment_jul2006/en/index.html (accessed July 12, 2010); Centers for Disease Control and Prevention, "CDC—Thimerosal FAQs—Vaccine Safety," www.cdc.gov/vaccine safety/Concerns/Thimerosal/thimerosal_faqs.html#3 (accessed July 12, 2010); Centers for Disease Control and Prevention, "CDC—Mercury and Thimerosal—Vaccine Safety," www.cdc.gov/vaccinesafety/Concerns/thimerosal/ (accessed July 12, 2010). For examples of some of the many papers that were produced showing no relationship between thimerosal and vaccines, see Thomas Verstraeten, Robert L. Davis, Frank DeStefano, Tracy A. Lieu, Philip H. Rhodes, Steven B. Black, Henry Shinefield, and Robert T. Chen, "Safety of Thimerosal-Containing Vaccines: A Two-Phased Study of Computerized Health Maintenance Organization Databases," *Pediatrics* 112 (2003): 1039–48; Anders Hviid, Michael Stellfeld, Jan Wohlfahrt, and Mads Melbye, "Association between Thimerosal-containing Vaccine and Autism," *Journal of the American Medical Association* 290 (2003): 1763–66; Paul Stehr-Green, Peet Tull, Michael Stellfeld, Preben-Bo Mortenson, and Diane Simpson, "Autism and Thimerosal-Containing Vaccines," *American Journal of Preventative Medicine* 25 (2003): 101–6; Kreesten M. Madsen, Marlene B. Lauritsen, Carsten B. Pedersen, Poul Thorsen, Anne-Marie Plesner, Peter H. Andersen, and Preben B. Mortensen, "Thimerosal and the Occurrence of Autism: Negative Ecological Evidence from Danish Population-Based Data," *Pediatrics* 112 (2003): 604–6; Nick Andres, Elizabeth Miller, Andrew Grant, Julia Stowe, Velda Osbourne, and Brent Taylor, "Thimerosal Exposure in Infants and Developmental Disorders: A Retrospective Cohort Study in the United Kingdom Does Not Support a Causal Association," *Pediatrics* 114 (2004): 584–91; Jon Heron, Jean Golding, and the ALSPAC Study Team, "Thimerosal Exposure in Infants and Developmental Disorders: A Prospective Cohort Study in the United Kingdom Does Not Support a Causal Association," *Pediatrics* 114 (2004): 577–83; Sarah K. Parker, Benjamin Schwartz, James Todd, and Larry K. Pickering, "Thimerosal-containing Vaccines and Autistic Spectrum Disorder: A Critical Review of the Published Original Data," *Pediatrics* 114 (2004): 793–804; Robert Schechter and Judith K. Grether, "Continuing Increases in Autism Reported to California's Developmental Services System: Mercury in Retrograde," *Archives of General Psychiatry* 65 (2008): 19–24; William W. Thompson, Cristofer Price, Barbara Goodson, David K. Shay, Patti Benson, Virginia L. Hinrichsen, Edwin Lewis, Eileen Eriksen, Paula Ray, S. Michael Marcy, John Dunn, Lisa A. Jackson, Tracy A. Lieu, Steve Black, Gerrie

Steward, Eric S. Weintraub, Robert L. Davis, and Frank DeStefano, "Early Thimerosal Exposure and Neuropsychological Outcomes at 7 to 10 Years," *The New England Journal of Medicine* 357 (2007): 1281–92. For examples of the scientific and medical communities' consensus on this issue, see Wendy Roberts and Mary Harford, "Immunization and Children at Risk for Autism," *Paediatric Child Health* 7 (November 2002): 623–32; Paul A. Offit and Rita K. Jew, "Addressing Parents' Concerns: Do Vaccines Contain Harmful Preservatives, Adjuvants, Additives, or Residuals?" *Pediatrics* 112 (2003): 1394–97; Michael G. Chez, Kathleen Chin, and Paul C. Hung, "Immunizations, Immunology, and Autism," *Seminars in Pediatric Neurology* 11 (2004): 214–17; Asif Doja and Wendy Roberts, "Immunizations and Autism: A Review of the Literature," *Canadian Journal of Neurological Sciences* 33 (2006): 341–46.

18. J. Zhang, "Clinical Observations in Ethyl Mercury Chloride Poisoning," *American Journal of Industrial Medicine* 5 (1984): 251–58; T. W. Clarkson, "The Pharmacology of Mercury Compounds," *Annual Review of Pharmacology* 12 (1971): 375–406; G. Lucier, "Ethyl and Methl Mercury: Pharmacokinetics and Toxicity," Transcript of the National Vaccine Advisory Committee Workshop on Thimerosal in Vaccines, Bethesda, Maryland (August 11, 1999); Ball et al., "An Assessment of Thimerosal Use in Childhood Vaccines," 1148–49; M. I. Hilmy, S. A. Rahim, and A. H. Abbas, "Norm and Lethal Mercury Levels in Human Beings," *Toxicology* 6 (1976): 155–59; Burbacher et al., "Comparison of Blood and Brain Mercury Levels," 1021. For examples of later studies, see Michael E. Pichichero, Angela Gentile, Norberto Giglio, Veronica Umido, Thomas Clarkson, Elsa Cernichiari, Grazyna Zareba, Carlos Gotelli, Mariana Gotelli, Lihan Yan, and John Treanor, "Mercury Levels in Newborns and Infants after Receipt of Thimerosal-containing Vaccines," *Pediatrics* 121 (2008): e208–e214. It should be noted that, in the details of the examinations of the literature on ethylmercury and methylmercury, I found a confusing difference in some of the claims. In their "Assessment of Thimerosal Use in Childhood Vaccines," Ball et al. explained, "Much of what we know about methylmercury toxicity comes from poisoning episodes in Japan, Iraq, the Seychelle Islands and the Faroe Islands. The Japanese case is the famous example from Minamata, Japan, from the 1950s and 1960s in which we first learned how mercury can bioaccumulate in aquatic systems and, when humans eat fish and shellfish that have high levels of mercury, they can be poisoned." The Japanese case clearly demonstrates that methylmercury is problematic. The authors make a similar claim about methylmercury with an example from Iraq in the 1970s in which mercury entered the food chain when farmers ignored authorities' warnings not to eat seed that had been treated with a fungicide manufactured by Dupont called Granoson M. Ball et al. claimed that Granoson M was a methylmercury fungicide. However, in a peer-reviewed article that appeared in the *Journal of Toxicology and Environmental Health* that was written by three people closely associated with the modern American anti-vaccination movement, they identified Granosan M as an ethylmercury-based fungicide. David A. Geier, Lisa K. Sykes, and Mark R. Geier, "A Review of Thimerosal (Merthiolate) and Its Ethylmercury Breakdown Product: Specific Historical Considerations Regarding Safety and Effectiveness," *Journal of Toxicology and Environmental Health, Part B* 10 (2007): 575–96. While I have reason to question Geier, Sykes, and Geier's claims based on their activism and involvement as professional experts in vaccine litigation, it seems that they are in fact correct. In subsequent research, I have found that it appears that

Ball et al. were incorrect in claiming that Granosan M was a methylmercury-based fungicide. In fact, it appears that Granosan M contains ethylmercury, which suggests that the information obtained from the Iraq example might be useful in helping us understand the harmful health effects of ethylmercury, which is the form of mercury found in thimerosal.

19. Ulrike Steurwald, Pal Weibe, Poul J. Jørgensen, Kristian Bjerve, John Brock, Birger Heinzow, Esben Budtz-Jørgensen, and Phillipe Grandjean, "Maternal Seafood Diet, Methylmercury Exposure, and Neonatal Neurologic Function," *Pediatrics* 136 (2000): 599–605; Pichichero, Cernichiari, Lopreiato, and Treanor, "Mercury Concentrations and Metabolism in Infants Receiving Vaccines Containing Thiomersal: A Descriptive Study," 1737–41; Burbacher, Shen, Liberato, Grant, Cernichiari, and Clarkson, "Comparison of Blood and Brain Mercury Levels in Infant Monkeys Exposed to Methylmercury or Vaccines Containing Thimerosal"; Centers for Disease Control and Prevention, "CDC—Thimerosal FAQs—Vaccine Safety," www.cdc.gov /vaccinesafety/Concerns/Thimerosal/thimerosal_faqs.html#4 (accessed July 13, 2010); Heron, Golding, and the ALSPAC Study Team, "Thimerosal Exposure in Infants and Developmental Disorders," 577.

20. Food and Drug Administration, "Letter to Manufacturers" (Washington, DC: Food and Drug Administration, 1999); "Notice to Readers: Thimerosal in Vaccines; A Joint Statement of the American Academy of Pediatrics and the Public Health Service," *Morbidity and Mortality Weekly Report* 48 (1999): 563–65; "Notice to Readers: Recommendations Regarding the Use of Vaccines that Contain Thimerosal as a Preservative," *Morbidity and Mortality Weekly Report* 48 (1999): 996–98; Neal A. Halsey, "Editorial: Limiting Infant Exposure to Thimerosal in Vaccines and Other Sources of Mercury," *Journal of the American Medical Association* 282 (1999): 1763–66.

21. American Academy of Pediatrics, "Vaccine Ingredients," www.aap.org/ immunization/families/ingredients.html#thimerosal (accessed July 13, 2010); Centers for Disease Control and Prevention, "CDC—Mercury and Thimerosal— Vaccine Safety," www.cdc.gov/vaccinesafety/Concerns/thimerosal/index.html (accessed July 13, 2010); Sandi Doughton, "State Lifts Limit on Mercury Preservative in Swine-Flu Shots," *The Seattle Times* (September 9, 2009). The story received over one hundred comments online, most of them quite critical of the Washington Health Department's decision.

22. See for example, Albert Enayati and Lyn Redwood, "Autism: A Unique Type of Mercury Poisoning," VaccinationNews.com, www.vaccinationnews.com/daily news/july2001/autismuniquemercpoison.htm (accessed July 13, 2010).

23. Offit, "A Cautionary Tale," 1279; Thomas W. Clarkson, Laszlo Magos, and Gary J. Myers, "The Toxicology of Mercury—Current Exposures and Clinical Manifestations," *New England Journal of Medicine* 349 (2003): 1736.

24. Evans Witt, "Birch Society Funds Movement for Laetrile," Associated Press October 10, 1977; Burton Goldberg, Larry Trivieri, John W. Anderson, *Alternative Medicine: The Definitive Guide*, 2nd ed. (Berkeley: Celestial Arts, 2002), 602; Allen, *Vaccine*, 392. Allen cites Beth Clay, author interview, May 2005, and Maurice Possley, "North Chicago Med School Sued on Cancer Cure," *Chicago Tribune*, July 29, 2004.

25. Aimee Howd, "When Vaccines Do Harm to Kids," www.gulfwarvets.com/ kids.htm (accessed July 13, 2010). Note the website hosting this story and how it demonstrates the correlation between advocacy for veterans with Gulf War Syndrome

and concerns about links between health problems and routine childhood vaccinations. Allen, *Vaccines,* 393.

26. Dan Burton, "Opening Statement, Committee on Government Reform, the Status of Research into Vaccine Safety and Autism," June 19, 2002, http://web.archive .org/web/20060316141931/http://ccmadoctors.ca/opening_statement_chairman_dan _b1.htm (accessed July 13, 2010).

27. Allen, *Vaccine,* 391; Dan Burton, "Opening Statement, Autism: Present Challenges, Future Needs—Why the Increased Rates?" Government Reform Committee, U.S. House of Representatives (April 6, 2000); Philip J. Hilts, "House Panel Asks for Study of a Vaccine," *New York Times,* April 7, 2000.

28. Arthur Allen, "The Not-So-Crackpot Autism Theory," *New York Times,* November 10, 2002; Orna Izakson, "Measuring Risk: Vaccines Save Lives, But Also Cause Health Problems," E. *The Environmental Magazine* (2003); Allen, *Vaccine,* 392. Brian Vastag, "Congressional Autism Hearings Continue: No Evidence MMR Vaccine Causes Disorder," *Journal of the American Medical Association* 285 (2001): 2567; Dan Burton, "Mercury in Medicine," *Congressional Record* (May 20, 2003): E1013.

29. Committee on Government Reform, U.S. House of Representatives, "Conflict of Interest in Vaccine Policy Making, Majority Staff Report, June 15, 2000."

30. Allen, *Vaccine,* 394; "Opinion: The Dan Burton Problem," *New York Times,* May 8, 1998; CNN, "Burton Draws Fire for Clinton 'Scumbag' Remark," April 22, 1998, www.cnn.com/ALLPOLITICS/1998/04/22/burton/ (accessed July 14, 2010); Don Van Natta Jr., "Panel Chief Refuses Apology to Clinton," April 22, 1998; "Rep. Burton Admits He Fathered a Son in an Affair," *New York Times,* September 5, 1998; "National News Brief: Burton Seeks Support after Admitting Affair," *New York Times,* September 6, 1998.

31. Christopher Beam, "Pig Pile: The Bizarre Alliance of the Far Left and the Far Right against Swine Flu Vaccinations," *Slate,* www.slate.com/id/2232187 (accessed July 22, 2010); Ryan Witt, "Video: Fight Erupts between MSNBC's Dr. Nancy and Rush Limbaugh over the H1N1 Vaccine," *Grand Rapids Examiner,* October 8, 2009; Media Matters for America, "Beck, Limbaugh Fomenting Fear about H1N1 Vaccine," http://mediamatters.org/print/research/200910070043 (accessed July 22, 2010); Bill O'Reilly, "Interview: Glenn Beck on H1N1 Flu Vaccine Mania," *Fox News,* www .foxnews.com/story/0,2933,563300,00.html (accessed July 22, 2010); Tara Parker-Pope, "Bill Maher vs. the Flu Vaccine," *New York Times,* October 13, 2009.

32. Verstraeten et al., "Safety of Thimerosal-containing Vaccines: A Two-Phased Study of Computerized Health Maintenance Organization Databases"; Robert F. Kennedy Jr., "Deadly Immunity: Robert F. Kennedy Investigates the Government Cover-up of a Mercury/Autism Scandal," *Rolling Stone,* June 20, 2005. For examples of how Simpsonwood is portrayed by anti-vaccinators, see "Simpsonwood Meeting on Mercury and Puerto Rico Meeting on Aluminum," www.autismhelpforyou.com/ Simpsonwood_And_Puerto percent20 percent20Rico.htm (accessed July 17, 2010); Safeminds, "Simpsonwood & Related Documents," www.safeminds.org/government -affairs/foia/simpsonwood.html (accessed July 17, 2010); Russell Blaylock, "The Truth Behind the Vaccine Cover-Up," www.wnho.net/vaccine_coverup.htm (accessed July 20, 2010).

33. Kennedy, "Deadly Immunity"; Committee on Government Reform, U.S. House of Representatives, "Hepatitis B Vaccine Hearings School Nurse Perspective:

Pattie White," May 17, 1999; Committee on Government Reform, U.S. House of Representatives, "Testimony by Boyd Haley," November 14, 2002; Institute of Medicine, Immunization Safety Review Committee, *Vaccines and Autism* (Washington DC: National Academies Press, 2004), 6–7. See also National Network for Immunization Information, "IOM Report on Vaccines and Autism," September 20, 2004, www.im munizationinfo.org/issues/iom-reports/iom-report-vaccines-and-autism (accessed July 22, 2010). In *Weiss v. Secretary of the Department of Health and Human Services*, Office of the Special Masters, U.S. Court of Federal Claims, October 9, 2003, Special Master Laura D. Millman wrote, "In other vaccine cases, Dr. Geier's testimony has similarly been accorded no weight. *Thompson v. Secretary of HHS*, No. 99-0436, 2003 WL 221439672 (Fed. Cl. Spec. Mstr. May 23, 2003); *Bruesewitz v. Secretary of HHS*, No. 95-0266, 2002 WL 3 1965744 (Fed. Cl. Spec. Mstr. Dec. 20,2002); *Raj v. Secretary of HHS*, No. 96-0294V, 2001 WL 963984, * 12 (Fed. Cl. Spec. Mstr. July 31, 2001); *Haim v. Secretary of HHS*, No. 90-1 03 lV, 1993 WL 346392 (Fed. Cl. Spec. Mstr. Aug. 27, 1993) ("Dr Geier's testimony is not reliable, or grounded in scientific methodology and procedure. His testimony is merely subjective belief and unsupported speculation."); *Marascalco v. Secretary of HHS*, No. 90-1571V, 1993 WL 277095 (Fed. Cl. Spec. Mstr. July 9, 1993) (where the special master described Dr. Geier's testimony as intellectually dishonest); *Einspahr v. Secretary of HHS*, No. 90-923V, 1992 WL 336396 (Cl. Ct. Spec. Mstr. Oct. 28, 1992), a, 17 F.3d 1444 (Fed. Cir. 1994); *Aldridge v. Secretary of HHS*, No. 90-2475V, 1992 WL 153770 (Cl. Ct. Spec. Mstr. June 11,1992); *Ormechea v. Secretary of HHS*, No. 90-1 683V, 1992 WL 15 18 16 (Cl. Ct. Spec. Mstr. June 10, 1992) ("Because Dr. Geier has made a profession of testifying in matters to which his professional background [obstetrics, genetics] is unrelated, his testimony is of limited value to the court."); *Daly v. Secretary of HHS*, No. 90-590V, 1991 WL 15473 (Cl. Ct. Spec. Mstr. July 26, 1991) ("The court is inclined not to allow Dr. Geier to testify before it on issues of Table injuries. Dr. Geier clearly lacks the expertise to evaluate the symptomatology of the Table injuries and render an opinion thereon.")." Numerous bloggers and pro-vaccine pundits have attacked the Geiers and their work. For example, see Stephen Barrett, "Dr. Mark Geier Severely Criticized," Casewatch.com, www.casewatch.org/civil/geier.shtml (accessed July 22, 2010); Confessions of a Quackbuster, "Mark Geier Untrustworthy: Autism, Thimerosal, Vaccinations," http:// quackfiles.blogspot.com/2005/03/mark-geier-untrustworthy-autism.html (accessed July 20, 2010); Mark R. Geier and David A. Geier, "Neurodevelopmental Disorders after Thimerosal-Containing Vaccines: A Brief Communication," *Experimental Biology and Medicine* 228 (2003): 660–64; Geier and Geier, "Pediatric MMR Vaccination Safety," *International Pediatrics* 18 (2003): 203–8; Geier and Geier, "Thimerosal in Childhood Vaccines, Neurodevelopment Disorders, and Heart Disease in the United States," *Journal of American Physicians and Surgeons* 8 (2003): 6–11; Jeff Bradstreet, David A. Geier, Jerold J. Kartzinel, James B. Adams, Mark R. Geier, "A Case-control Study of Mercury Burden in Children with Autistic Spectrum Disorders," *Journal of American Physicians and Surgeons* 8 (2003): 76–79; Geier and Geier, "An Assessment of the Impact of Thimerosal on Neurodevelopmental Disorders," *Pediatric Rehabilitation* 6 (2003): 97–102; Geier and Geier, "A Comparative Evaluation of the Effects of MMR Immunization and Mercury Doses from Thimerosal-containing Childhood Vaccines on the Population Prevalence of Autism," *Medical Science Monitor* 10 (2004): 33–39; Geier and Geier, "The Potential Importance of Steroids in the

Treatment of Autistic Spectrum Disorders," *Medical Hypothesis* 64 (2005): 946–54; Geier and Geier, "Neurodevelopmental Disorders Following Thimerosal-containing Childhood Immunizations"; Geier and Geier, "A Two-Phased Population Epidemiological Study of the Safety of Thimerosal-Containing Vaccines: A Follow-Up Analysis," *Medical Science Monitor* 11 (2005): 160–70; Geier and Geier, "An Evaluation of the Effects of Thimerosal on Neurodevelopmental Disorders Reported Following DTP and Hib Vaccines in Comparison to DTPH Vaccine in the United States," *Journal of Toxicology and Environmental Health* 69 (2006): 1481–95; Geier and Geier, "Early Downward Trends in Neurodevelopmental Disorders Following Removal of Thimerosal-Containing Vaccine," *Journal of American Physicians and Surgeons* 11 (2006): 8–13; Gardiner Harris and Anahad O'Connor, "On Autism's Cause, It's Parents vs. Research," *New York Times*, June 25, 2005; Arthur Allen, "Sticking Up for Thimerosal: Read the Studies—It's Safe," *Slate*, August 2, 2005. For the corrections to Kennedy's article, see www.rollingstone.com/politics/story/7395411/deadly_immu nity/print (accessed July 20, 2010).

34. *The Daily Show with Jon Stewart*, July 20, 2005.

35. Union of Concerned Scientists, "Scientific Integrity in Policymaking: An Investigation into the Bush Administration's Misuse of Science" (Cambridge, MA: Union of Concerned Scientists, 2004), 1. Examples of criticisms of the Bush administration for inappropriately politicizing science can be found in Anne C. Mulkern, "When Advocates Become Regulators," *Denver Post*, May 23, 2004; Chris Mooney, *The Republican War on Science* (New York: Basic Books, 2006); Oreskes and Conway, *Merchants of Doubt*; John F. Kennedy Jr., *Crimes Against Nature: How George W. Bush & His Corporate Pals are Plundering the Country & Hijacking Our Democracy* (New York: Harper Perennial, 2005); Michael Specter, *Denialism: How Irrational Thinking Hinders Science* (New York: Penguin Press, 2009); *The Daily Show with Jon Stewart*, July 20, 2005; Amy Wallace, "An Epidemic of Fear: How Panicked Parents Skipping Shots Endangers Us All," *Wired*, November 2009, 129–35, 166–70; "Rants: The War on Science," *Wired*, January 2010, 16–17.

36. Virginia Hughes, "Mercury Rising," *Nature Medicine* 13 (2007): 896–97; Harris and O'Connor, "On Autism's Cause, It's Parents vs. Research." Offit, *Autism's False Prophets*, xi–xviii.

37. Harris and O'Connor, "On Autism's Cause, It's Parents vs. Research."

CHAPTER 4: MMR and Autism

1. "Parents Left Stunned as MMR Doctor Is Forced Out," *Telegraph,* February 12, 2001.

2. A. J. Wakefield, A. M. Sawyerr, A. P. Dhillon, R. M. Pittilo, P. M. Rowles, A. A. M. Lewis, and Roy E. Pounder, "Pathogenesis of Crohn's Disease," *Lancet* (1989): 1057–62; A. J. Wakefield, E. A. Sankey, A. P. Dillon, A. M. Sawyerr, L. More, R. Sin, R. M. Pittilo, P. M. Rowles, M. Hudson, and A. A. Lewis, et al., "Granulomatous Vasculitis in Crohn's Disease," *Journal of Gastroenterology* 100 (1990): 1279–87.

3. Kary Mullis, "The Unusual Origin of the Polymerase Chain Reaction," *Scientific American* 262 (1990): 56–61, 64–65.

4. G. W. Farmer, M. V. Monroe, D. A. Fuccillo, L. H. Barbosa, S. Ritman, J. L. Serer, and G. L. Gitnick, "Viral Investigations in Ulcerative Colitis and Regional

Enteritis," *Journal of Gastroenterology* 65 (1973): 8–18; H. S. Cooper, E. C. Raffensper, and L. Jonas, "Cytomegalovirus Inclusions in Patients with Ulcerative Colitis and Toxic Dilation Requiring Colonic Resection," *Journal of Gastroenterology* 72 (1977): 1253–56; S. Sidi, J. H. Graham, S. A. Razvi, and P. A. Banks, "Cytomegalovirus Infection of the Colon Associated with Ulcerative Colitis," *Archives of Surgery* 114 (1979): 857–59; T. Berk, S. J. Gordon, and H. Y. Choi, "Cytomegalovirus Infection of the Colon: A Possible Role in Exacerbation of Inflammatory Bowel Disease," *Journal of Gastroenterology* 80 (1985): 355–60; A. H. M. Span, W. Mullers, A. M. M. Miltenburg, and C. A. Bruggerman, "Cytomegalovirus Induced PMN Adherence in Relation to an ELAM-1 Antigen Present on Infected Endothelial Cell Monolayers," *Immunology* 72 (1991): 355–60; R. R. MacGregor, H. M. Friedman, and E. J. Macarack, "Virus Infection of Endothelial Cells Increases Granulocyte Adherence," *Journal of Clinical Investigation* 65 (1980): 1469–77; T. Matsumoto, A. Ritano, S. Nakamura, N. Oshitani, A. Obata, M. Hiki, H. Hashimura, K. Okawa, K. Kobayashi, and H. Nagura, "Possible Role of Vacular Endothelial Cells in Immune Responses in Colonic Mucosa Examine Immunocytochemically in Subjects with and without Ulcerative Colitis," *Clinical and Experimental Immunology* 78 (1989): 424–30; C. O. Elson, "The Immunology of Inflammatory Bowel Disease," in *Inflammatory Bowel Disease*, ed. J. B. Kirsner and R. G. Shorter, 3rd ed. (Philadelphia: Lea and Febiger, 1988), vol. 7, 97–174.

5. Andrew J. Wakefield, J. D. Fox, A. M. Sawyerr, J. E. Taylor, C. H. Sweenie, M. Smith, V. C. Emery, M. Hudson, R. S. Tedder, and Roy E. Pounder, "Detection of Herpesvirus DNA in the Large Intestine of Patients with Ulcerative Colitis and Crohn's Disease Using the Nested Polymerase Chain Reaction," *Journal of Medical Virology* 38 (1992): 183–90; John Walker-Smith, *Enduring Memories: A Paediatric Gastroenterologist Remembers; A Tale of London and Sydney* (Spennymoor: The Memoir Club, 2003), 241; E. Stubbs, "Autistic Symptoms in a Child with Congenital Cytomegalovirus Infection," *Journal of Autism and Childhood Schizophrenia* 8 (1978): 37–43; P. Markowitz, "Autism in a Child with Cytomegalovirus Infection," *Journal of Autism and Developmental Disorders* 13 (1983): 249–53; S. A. Ivarsson, I. Bierre, P. Veofors, and K. Ahlfors, "Autism as One of Several Disabilities in Two Children with Congenital Cytomegalovirus Infection," *Neuropediatrics* 21 (1990): 102–3; G. Delong, S. Beau, and F. Brown, "Acquired Reversible Autistic Syndrome in Acute Encephalophatic Illness in Children," *Archives of Neurology* 38 (1981): 191–94; C. Gillberg, "Onset at Age 14 of Typical Autistic Syndrome: A Case Report of a Previously Normal Girl with Herpes Encephalitis," *Journal of Autism and Development Disorders* 14 (1986): 1–8; M. Ghaziuddin, L. Y. Tsai, L. Eileirs, and N. Ghaziuddin, "Brief Report: Autism and Herpes Simplex Encephalitis," *Journal of Autism and Development Disorders* 22 (1992): 107–13.

6. Andrew J. Wakefield, R. M. Pittilo, R. Sim, S. L. Cosby, J. R. Stephenson, A. P. Dhillon, and Roy E. Pounder, "Evidence of Persistent Measles Virus Infection in Crohn's Disease," *Journal of Medical Virology* 39 (1993): 345–53.

7. Masahiro Iizuka, Osumu Nakagomi, Mitsuro Chiba, Shigeharu Ueda, and Osamu Masamune, "Absence of Measles Virus in Crohn's Disease," *Lancet* 345 (1995): 199; Y. Haga, O. Funakoshi, K. Kuroe, L. Kanazawa, H. Nakajima, H. Saito, Y. Murata, A. Munakata, and Y. Yoshida, "Absence of Measles Viral Genomic Sequence in Intestinal Tissues from Crohn's Disease by Nested Polymerase Chain Reaction," *Gut* 38 (1996): 211–15.

8. A. Ekbom, A. J. Wakefield, M. Zack, and H. O. Adami, "Potential Measles Infection and Subsequent Crohn's Disease," *Lancet* 344 (1994): 508–10; Anders Ekbom, Peter Daszak, Wolfgang Kraaz, and Andrew J. Wakefield, "Crohn's Disease after In-Utero Measles Virus Exposure," *Lancet* 348 (1996): 515–17.

9. Andrew J. Wakefield, Anders Ekbom, Amar P. Dhillon, R. Michael Pittilo, and Roy E. Pounder, "Crohn's Disease: Pathogenesis and Persistent Measles Virus Infection," *Journal of Gastroenterology* 108 (1995): 911–16.

10. N. P. Thompson, S. M. Montgomery, R. E. Pounder, and A. J. Wakefield, "Is Measles Vaccination a Risk Factor for Inflammatory Bowel Disease?" *Lancet* 345 (1995): 1071–74.

11. Peter A. Patriarca and Judy A. Beeler, "Measles Vaccination and Inflammatory Bowel Disease," *Lancet* 345 (1995): 1062–63.

12. Paddy Farrington and Elizabeth Miller, "Letters to the Editor: Measles Vaccination as a Risk Factor of Inflammatory Bowel Disease," *Lancet* 345 (1995): 1362; K. C. Calman, "Letters to the Editor: Measles Vaccination as a Risk Factor of Inflammatory Bowel Disease," *Lancet* 345 (1995): 1362; Philip D. Minor, "Letters to the Editor: Measles Vaccination as a Risk Factor of Inflammatory Bowel Disease," *Lancet* 345 (1995): 1362–63; Thomas T. MacDonald, "Letters to the Editor: Measles Vaccination as a Risk Factor of Inflammatory Bowel Disease," *Lancet* 345 (1995): 1363; David Miller and Adrian Renton, "Letters to the Editor: Measles Vaccination as a Risk Factor of Inflammatory Bowel Disease," *Lancet* 345 (1995): 1363; Tony Baxter and John Radford, "Letters to the Editor: Measles Vaccination as a Risk Factor of Inflammatory Bowel Disease," *Lancet* 345 (1995): 1363.

13. Calman, "Letters to the Editor," 1362. On Calman's response to the public concerns about the MMR vaccine that emerged in 1998, see BBC News, "MMR Leaflets Seek to Reassure Parents" (September 4, 1998). Andrew J. Wakefield, *Callous Disregard: Autism and Vaccines; The Truth behind a Tragedy* (New York: Skyhorse Publishing, 2010), 54. Wakefield cites for this quote a letter from Zuckerman to Calman dated January 22, 1997. Baxter and Radford, "Letters to the Editor," 1363.

14. J. Hermon-Taylor, J. For, N. Sumar, D. Millar, T. Doran, and M. Tizard, "Letters to the Editor: Measles Virus and Crohn's Disease," *Lancet* 345 (1995): 922. The paper they cited was Wakefield et al., "Evidence of Persistent Measles Virus Infection in Crohn's Disease," 345–63; Angus Nicoll, David Elliman, and Euan Ross, "MMR Vaccinations and Autism 1998," *British Medical Journal* 316 (1998): 715–16.

15. Walker-Smith, *Enduring Memories*, 241–42; Richard Horton, "Correspondence: Autism, Inflammatory Bowel Disease, and MMR Vaccine," *Lancet* 351 (1998): 908–9; Nick P. Thompson, S. M. Montgomery, Roy E. Pounder, and Andrew J. Wakefield, "Letters to the Editor: Measles Vaccination as a Risk Factor for Inflammatory Bowel Disease, Authors' Reply," *Lancet* 345 (1995): 1364.

16. Nick P. Thompson, Douglas M. Fleming, Roy E. Pounder, and Andrew J. Wakefield, "Letter to the Editor: Crohn's Disease, Measles, and Measles Vaccination; A Case-Control Failure," *Lancet* 347 (1996): 263; Mark Feeney, Andrew Clegg, Paul Winwood, and Jonathon Snook, "A Case-Control Study of Measles Vaccination and Inflammatory Bowel Disease," *Lancet* 350 (1997): 764–66.

17. Scott M. Montgomery, D. L. Morris, R. E. Pounder, and A. J. Wakefield, "Correspondence: Measles Vaccination and Inflammatory Bowel Disease," *Lancet* 350 (1997): 1774; Mark Feeney, Andrew Clegg, Paul Winwood, and Jonathon Snook,

"Correspondence: Measles Vaccination and Inflammatory Bowel Disease, Authors' Reply," *Lancet* 350 (1997): 1774; Wim Van Damme, Lut Lynen, Guy Kegels, and Wim Van Leberghe, "Correspondence: Measles Vaccination and Inflammatory Bowel Disease," *Lancet* 350 (1997): 1774–75; and Masahiro Iizuka and Osamu Masamune, "Correspondence: Measles Vaccination and Inflammatory Bowel Disease," *Lancet* 350 (1997): 1775; Nicholas Chadwick, Ian J. Bruce, Silke Schepelmann, Roy E. Pounder, and Andrew J. Wakefield, "Measles Virus RNA Is Not Detected in Inflammatory Bowel Disease Using Hybrid Capture and Reverse Transcription Followed by the Polymerase Chain Reaction," *Journal of Medical Virology* 55 (1998): 305–11.

18. Jane Medcalf, "Editorial: Is Measles Infection Associated with Crohn's Disease?" *British Medical Journal* 316 (1998): 166; World Health Organization, Expanded Programme on Immunization, "Association Between Measles Infection and the Occurrence of Chronic Inflammatory Bowel Disease," *Weekly Epidemiological Record* 73 (1998): 33–39.

19. Walker-Smith, *Enduring Memories*, 241.

20. Andrew J. Wakefield, Simon H. Murch, A. Anthony, John Linnell, D. M. Casson, M. Malik, Mark Berelowitz, A. P. Dhillon, Michael A. Thomson, P. Harvey, A. Valentine, S. E. Davies, and John A. Walker-Smith, "Ileal-Lymphoid-Nodular Hyperplasia, Non-specific Colitis, and Pervasive Developmental Disorder in Children," *Lancet* 351 (1998): 637–41.

21. Hans Asperger, "Die Psychopathologie des Coeliakakranken Kindes," *Annales Paediatrici* 197 (1961): 146–51; Walker-Smith, *Enduring Memories*, 238; Wakefield et al., "Ileal-Lymphoid-Nodular Hyperplasia, Non-Specific Colitis, and Pervasive Developmental Disorder in Children," 640; Panksepp, "A Neurochemical Theory of Autism," *Trends in Neurosciences* 2 (1979): 174–77; K. L. Reichelt, K. Hole, A. Hamberger, G. Saelid, P. D. Edminison, C. B. Braestrup, O. Lingjaerde, P. Ledaal, and H. Orbeck, "Biologically Active Peptide-containing Fractions in Schizophrenia and Childhood Autism," *Advances in Biochemical Psychopharmacology* 28 (1993): 627–43. P. Shattock, A. Kennedy, F. Rowell, and T. P. Berney, "Role of Neuropeptides in Autism and Their Relationships with Classical Neurotransmitters," *Brain Dysfunction* 3 (1991): 328–45; Wakefield et al., "Ileal-Lymphoid-Nodular Hyperplasia, Non-Specific Colitis, and Pervasive Developmental Disorder in Children," 641.

22. Richard Horton, *Second Opinion: Doctor's Diseases and Decisions in Modern Medicine* (London: Granta Publications, 2003), 208; Wakefield et al., "Ileal-Lymphoid-Nodular Hyperplasia, Non-Specific Colitis, and Pervasive Developmental Disorder in Children," 641; Royal Free Hospital School of Medicine, "Press Release: New Research Links Autism and Bowel Disease," http://briandeer.com/mmr/royal-free-press-1998.pdf (accessed July 1, 2008).

23. Walker-Smith, *Enduring Memories*, 242; Wakefield, *Callous Disregard*, 84–85.

24. M. A. Afzal, P. D. Minor, J. Begley, M. L. Bentley, E. Armitage, S. Ghosh, and A. Ferguson, "Absence of Measles-Virus Genome in Inflammatory Bowel Disease," *Lancet* 351 (1998): 646–47. Later that year, Wakefield coauthored a paper with two colleagues in the Inflammatory Bowel Disease Study Group at the Royal Free Hospital in London and another researcher from the University of Greenwich in London that reported that they had also failed to find any measles virus RNA in tissue samples taken from patients with inflammatory bowel disease. Nicholas Chadwick, Ian J. Bruce, Silke Schepelmann, Roy E. Pounder, and Andrew J. Wakefield, "Measles

Virus RNA Is Not Detected in Inflammatory Bowel Disease Using Hybrid Capture and Reverse Transcription Followed by the Polymerase Chain Reaction," *Journal of Medical Virology* 55 (1998): 305–11.

25. Robert T. Chen and Frank DeStefano, "Vaccine Adverse Events: Causal or Coincidental?" *Lancet* 351 (1998): 611–12.

26. Chen and DeStefano, "Vaccine Adverse Events," 611–12.

27. J. W. Lee, B. Melgaard, C. J. Clements, M. Kane, E. K. Mulholland, and J-M. Olivé, "Correspondence: Autism, Inflammatory Bowel Disease, and MMR Vaccine," *Lancet* 351 (1998): 905; David Black, Henry Prempeh, and Tony Baxter, "Correspondence: Autism, Inflammatory Bowel Disease, and MMR Vaccine," *Lancet* 351 (1998): 905–6; A. J. Beale, "Correspondence: Autism, Inflammatory Bowel Disease, and MMR Vaccine," *Lancet* 351 (1998): 906; Sarah J. O'Brien, Ian G. Jones, and Peter Christie, "Correspondence: Autism, Inflammatory Bowel Disease, and MMR Vaccine," *Lancet* 351 (1998): 906; Keith J. Lindley and Peter J. Milla, "Correspondence: Autism, Inflammatory Bowel Disease, and MMR Vaccine," *Lancet* 351 (1998): 907.

28. Andrew J. Wakefield, "Correspondence: Autism, Inflammatory Bowel Disease, and MMR Vaccine," *Lancet* 351 (1998): 908.

29. Simon Murch, Mike Thomson, and John Walker-Smith, "Correspondence: Autism, Inflammatory Bowel Disease, and MMR Vaccine," *Lancet* 351 (1998): 908; Walker-Smith, *Enduring Memories*, 241.

30. Horton, "Correspondence," 908–9; Horton, *Second Opinions*, 213–14.

31. A. Rouse, "Correspondence: Inflammatory Bowel Disease, and MMR Vaccine," *Lancet* 351 (1998): 1356; Andrew J. Wakefield, "Correspondence: Inflammatory Bowel Disease, and MMR Vaccine," *Lancet* 351 (1998): 1356; Wakefield, "Correspondence," 1356; M. A. Tettenborn, "Correspondence: Inflammatory Bowel Disease, and MMR Vaccine," *Lancet* 351 (1998): 1357.

32. "National Vaccine Information Center (NVIC)—About Us," www.909shot.com/About.htm (accessed July 3, 2008); Barbara Loe Fisher, "Correspondence: Inflammatory Bowel Disease, and MMR Vaccine," *Lancet* 351 (1998): 1357–58.

33. Thompson et al., "Is Measles Vaccination a Risk Factor for Inflammatory Bowel Disease?" 1072; Wakefield, *Callous Disregard*, 85.

34. Naomi Rogers, *Dirt and Disease: Polio Before FDR* (New Brunswick: Rutgers University Press, 1992).

35. Wakefield and Montgomery cited Vijendra K. Singh, S. X. Lin, and V. C. Yang, "Serological Association of Measles Virus and Human Herpesvirus-6 with Brain Autoantibodies in Autism," *Clinical Immunology and Immunopathology* 89 (1998): 105–8.

36. Ann-Mari Knivsberg, Kari Wigg, G Lind, and K. Reichelt, "Dietary Intervention in Autistic Children," *Brain Dysfunction* 3 (1990): 315–17; Andrew J. Wakefield and Scott M. Montgomery, "Autism, Viral Infections and Measles-Mumps-Rubella Vaccination," *Israeli Medical Association Journal* 1 (1999): 183–87.

37. These studies were M. A. Afzal, P. D. Minor, J. Begley, M. L. Bently, E. Armitage, S. Ghosh, and A. Fergusan, "Absence of Measles-Virus Genome in Inflammatory Bowel Disease," *Lancet* 351 (1998): 646–47; Hisahi Kawashima, Takayuki Mori, Yasuyo Kashiwagi, Kouju Takekuma, Akinori Hoshika, and Andrew Wakefield, "Detection and Sequencing of Measles Virus from Peripheral Mononuclear Cells from Patients with Inflammatory Bowel Disease and Autism," *Digestive Diseases and*

Sciences 45 (2000): 723–29; Masahiro Iizuka, Hiroaki Itou, Mitsuro Chiba, Tomoyuki Shirasaka, and Sumio Watanabe, "Correspondence: The MMR Question," *Lancet* 356 (2000): 160–61.

38. Andrew J. Wakefield and Scott M. Montgomery, "Measles Virus as a Risk for Inflammatory Bowel Disease: An Unusually Tolerant Approach," *American Journal of Gastroenterology* 95 (2000): 1389–92; Andrew J. Wakefield, A. Anthony, S. H. Murch, M. Thomson, Scott M. Montgomery, S. Davies, J. J. O'Leary, M. Berelowitz, and John A. Walker-Smith, "Enterocolitis in Children with Developmental Disorders," *American Journal of Gastroenterology* 95 (2000): 2285–95; Eamonn M. M. Quigley and David Hurley, "Autism and the Gastrointestinal Tract," *American Journal of Gastroenterology* 95 (2000): 2154–56.

39. Theodore Heller, "Uber Dementia Infantilis: Verblödungsprozeß im Kindesalter," *Zeitschrift für die Erforschung und Behandlung des Jugendlichen Schwachsinns* 2 (1908): 17–28; Wakefield, *Callous Disregard*, 134–40; Sears, *The Autism Book*, 6–7.

40. Brent Taylor, Elizabeth Miller, C. Paddy Farrington, Maria-Christina Petropoulos, Isabelle Favot-Mayaud, Jun Li, and Pauline A. Waight, "Autism and Measles, Mumps, and Rubella Vaccine: No Epidemiological Evidence for a Causal Association," *Lancet* 353 (1999): 2026–29.

41. Frank DeStefano and Robert T. Chen, "Commentary: Negative Association between MMR and Autism," *Lancet* 353 (1999): 1987–88.

42. Committee on Safety of Medicines, "The Safety of MMR Vaccine," *Current Problems in Pharmacovigilance* 25 (1999): 9–11.

43. Neal A. Halsey Susan Hyman, and the Conference Writing Panel, "Measles-Mumps-Rubella Vaccine and Autistic Spectrum Disorder: Report from the New Challenges in Childhood Immunizations Conference Convened in Oak Brook, Illinois, June 12–13, 2000," *Pediatrics* 107 (2001): E84, www.pediatrics.org/cgi/content/full/107/5/e84 (accessed July 8, 2009).

44. The MRC report cited Wakefield et al., "Ileal-Lymphoid-Nodular Hyperplasia, Non-specific Colitis, and Pervasive Developmental Disorder in Children." Kawashima, et al., "Detection and Sequencing of Measles Virus from Peripheral Mononuclear Cells from Patients with Inflammatory Bowel Disease and Autism." Singh, et al., "Antibodies to Myelin Basic Protein in Children with Autistic Behavior"; Singh et al., "Serological Association of Measles Virus and Human Herpesvirus-6 with Brain Autoantibodies in Autism"; Halsey and Hyman, "Measles-Mumps-Rubella Vaccine and Autistic Spectrum Disorder: Report from the New Challenges in Childhood Immunizations Conference Convened in Oak Brook, Illinois, June 12–13, 2000," *Pediatrics* 107 (2001): E84; Medical Research Council, "Review of Autism Research: Epidemiology and Causes," December 2001.

45. Kreesten Meldgaard Madsen, Anders Hviid, Mogens Vestergaard, Diana Schendel, Jan Wohlfahrt, Poul Thorsen, Jørn Olsen, and Mads Melbye, "A Population-Based Study of Measles, Mumps, and Rubella Vaccination and Autism," *New England Journal of Medicine* 347 (2002): 1477–82.

46. Brian Deer, who came to be one of the most aggressive critics of Wakefield, has published the transcript of the interview with Wakefield on his website. Brian Deer, "Brian Deer Investigates MMR—Royal Free Hospital Video," http://briandeer.com/wakefield/royal-video.htm (accessed June 11, 2010); "Parents Left Stunned as MMR Doctor Is Forced Out," *Telegraph,* February 12, 2001.

47. Wakefield and Montgomery, "Autism, Viral Infection and Measles-Mumps-Rubella Vaccination," 185. In support of this claim they cite Deykin and MacMahon, "Viral Exposure and Autism," *American Journal of Epidemiology* 109, no. 66 (1979): 28–38.

48. "Getting the Facts Straight on MMR," *Pulse*, June 26, 1999, 77.

49. "Sarah Dean," www.arete4life.co.uk/profiles/sarah-dean (accessed June 19, 2008); Stephen Hayward, "MMR Jab Snub for Minister," *Sunday Mirror*, February 17, 2002; Jeremy Laurance, "MMR Fears Lead to Big Demand for Separate Jabs," *Independent* (London), February 22, 2003; "Sixty Children Get Single Measles Vaccine Despite War of Words," *Waterford News & Star*, December 6, 2002; Christine Doyle, "Real Security Is a Single Jab," *Telegraph*, February 5, 2002. Information about Direct Health 2000's services can be found on their website, www.dh2.co.uk. (accessed July 11, 2008).

50. Jeremy Laurance, "MMR Fears Lead to Big Demand for Separate Jabs," *Independent*, February 22, 2003; Jeremy Laurance, "MMR Vaccines: Are Three Jabs Really Better than One?" *Independent*, January 18, 2001; "Sixty Children Get Single Measles Vaccine Despite War of Words," *Waterford News & Star*, December 6, 2002; "Safety Fears Voiced as British Company Offers Single Vaccines," *Waterford News & Star*, June 3, 2005.

51. Jenny Hope, "Doctors' Children Avoid MMR," *Daily Mail*, May 1, 2003; Doyle, "Real Security Is a Single Jab."

52. To determine whether a newspaper was oriented toward the Labor Party or the Conservative Party, I relied on a Ipsos MORI survey from 2004, which asked 21,727 British adults about their voting intentions and the newspapers they typically read. Ipsos MORI, "Voting Intention by Newspaper Readership Quarter 1 2005," www.ipsos-mori.com/researchpublications/researcharchive/poll.aspx?oItemId=580&view=wide (accessed June 11, 2010).

53. Medical Research Council, "Review of Autism Research: Epidemiology and Causes" (December 2001); Lorraine Fraser, "Studies Fail to Disprove Autism Link to MMR Jab," *Telegraph*, September 12, 2001. Additional stories in the *Telegraph* that show a bias in favor of Wakefield include Lorraine Fraser, "Revealed: More Evidence to Challenge the Safety of MMR," *Telegraph*, June 16, 2002; Lorraine Fraser, "US Experts Back MMR Doctor's Findings," *Telegraph*, June 23, 2002; BBC News, "Study Backs Safety of MMR Vaccine," September 9, 2004, http://news.bbc.co.uk/go/pr/fr/-/2/hi/health/3640898.stm (accessed June 24, 2008).

54. Jeremy Laurance, "MMR Vaccines: Are Three Jabs Really Better Than One?" *Independent*, January 18, 2001.

55. Benedict Brogan, "Come Clean on MMR, Labour MP Tells Blair," *Telegraph*, December 22, 2001; Lorraine Fraser, "Blair Hints that Leo had MMR Jab as Vaccine Rebellion Mounts," *Telegraph*, December 23, 2001; Benedict Brogan, "Pressure Mounts on Blair To Say if Leo Had MMR Jab," *Telegraph*, December 23, 2001. According to a 2004 survey by Ipsos MORI that reported on newspaper readers' voting intentions, 53 percent of the regular readers of the *Daily Mail* intended to vote for the Conservative Party, while only 21 percent planned to vote for the Labour Party. The *Daily Mail* had the second highest proportion of Conservative Party-voting readings of all U.K. papers. Only the *Daily Telegraph* was higher. Ipsos MORI, "Voting Intention by Newspaper Readership," www.ipsos-mori.com/copnent/voting-intention-by

-newspaper-readership.ashx. (accessed June 20, 2008). See also Caroline White, "Open Season on MMR," *British Medical Journal* (2002): 120.

56. White, "Open Season on MMR," 120; Horton, *Second Opinions*, 216.

57. Andrew Wakefield, "Why I Owe It to Parents to Question Triple Vaccine," *Sunday Herald*, February 10, 2002.

58. Brian Deer, "MMR Scare Doctor Faces List of Charges," *Sunday Times*, September 11, 2005; Lorraine Fraser, "Anti-MMR Doctor Is Forced Out," *Telegraph*, February 12, 2001.

59. Brian Deer, "Revealed: MRR Research Scandal," *Sunday Times*, February 22, 2004.

60. Wakefield, *Callous Disregard*, 106; Horton, *MMR*, 3, 48–53.

61. "A Statement by the Royal Free and University College Medical School and the Royal Free Hampstead NHS Trust," *Lancet* 363 (March 6 2004): 824; "A Statement by the Editors of *The Lancet*," *Lancet* 363 (March 6, 2004), 820–21. Wakefield wrote that Deer's presentation was three hours long. Horton, who was present at it, wrote that it was five hours long. Wakefield, *Callous Disregard*, 106; Horton, *MMR*, 3; Wakefield, *Callous Disregard*, 101–14, 124.

62. "About COPE," www.publicationethics.org.uk/about (accessed June 6, 2008); Richard Horton, "A Statement by the Editors of *The Lancet*," *Lancet* 363 (2004): 820–21.

63. Simon H. Murch, Andrew Anthony, David H. Casson, Mohsin Malik, Mark Berelowitz, Amar P. Dhillon, Michael A. Thomson, Alan Valentine, Susan E. Davies, and John A. Walker-Smith, "Retraction of an Interpretation," *Lancet* 363 (March 6, 2004): 750.

64. Taylor et al., "Autism and Measles, Mumps, and Rubella Vaccine," 2026–29; Committee on Safety of Medicines, "The Safety of MMR Vaccine," 9–11; Andrew J. Wakefield, "Correspondence: MMR Vaccination and Autism," *Lancet* 354 (1999): 949–50.

65. V. Demicheli, T. Jefferson, A. Rivetti, and D. Price, "Vaccines for Measles, Mumps and Rubella in Children," *Cochrane Database of Systematic Reviews* (2005).

66. The Cochrane Library, "The Cochrane Library Publishes the Most Thorough Survey of MMR Vaccination Data Which Strongly Supports Its Use" (October 19, 2005), www.cochrane.org/press/MMR_final.pdf (accessed June 18, 2008).

67. Melanie Phillips, "MMR: The Unanswered Questions," *Daily Mail*, October 31, 2005; Michael Fitzpatrick, "Why Can't the *Daily Mail* Eat Humble Pie over MMR?" *British Medical Journal* 331 (November 12, 2005): 1148.

68. Thoughtful House Center for Children, "Annual Report, 2007," www.thoughtfulhouse.org/annual-report-2007.pdf (accessed June 12, 2010).

69. Sarah Boseley, "Andrew Wakefield Found 'Irresponsible' by GMC over MMR Vaccine Scare," *Guardian*, January 28, 2010; Raf Sanchez and David Rose, "Dr. Andrew Wakefield Struck off Medical Register," *Times*, May 25, 2010; Wakefield, *Callous Disregard*, 177.

CHAPTER 5: Science and the Celebrity

1. *The Daily Show with Jon Stewart*, July 20, 2005; Andrew J. Wakefield, *Callous Disregard: Autism and Vaccines; The Truth behind a Tragedy* (New York: Skyhorse Publishing, 2010), 5.

2. An excellent example of how public controversies over scientific subjects can be initiated or perpetuated by a small number of oppositional critics can be found in Naomi Oreskes and Erik M. Conway, *Merchants of Doubt: How a Handful of Scientists Obscured the Truth about Issues from Tobacco Smoke to Global Warming* (New York: Bloomsbury Press, 2010). For a discussion of how minority groups can take advantage of limitations of their minority position to influence a political system, see James C. Scott, *Weapons of the Weak: Everyday Forms of Peasant Resistance* (New Haven: Yale University Press, 1985); Richard Horton, "Heart vs. Head: The Issue of MMR Rather than Single Vaccines Is Not Going to Go Away Anytime Soon," *Guardian*, April 24, 2006.

3. "Parents Still Fear Autism Could Be Linked to Vaccines, Poll Shows," *Science Daily*, October 4, 2008, www.sciencedaily.com/releases/2008/10/081003122536.htm (accessed December 19, 2008). The most recent survey reported that 25 percent of American parents believe that "some vaccines cause autism in healthy children." Gary L. Freed, Sarah J. Clark, Amy T. Butchart, Diane C. Singer, and Matthew M. Davis, "Parental Vaccine Concerns in 2009," *Pediatrics* 125 (2010): 656.

4. "Editorial: On Message, Off Target; Official Advice on Vaccination is Too Often Poorly Transmitted," *Nature* 452 (2008): 128.

5. Jake Tapper, comment on "John McCain Enters the Autism Wars," *Political Punch Blog*, posted February 29, 2008, http://blogs.abcnews.com/politicalpunch/2008/02/john-mccain-ent.html (accessed July 21, 2008); "Dr. Obama and Dr. McCain," *Fact Checker Blog*, posted April 22, 2008, http://blog.washingtonpost.com/fact-checker/2008/04/dr_obama_and_dr_mccain.html (accessed July 21, 2008); Lila Guterman, "John McCain's Autism Comment Prompts Outrage in the Blogosphere," *Chronicle of Higher Education*, http://chronicle.com/blogs/election/1794 (accessed, July 7, 2009); Benedict Carey, "Into the Fray Over the Cause of Autism," *New York Times*, March 4, 2008.

6. Collin Gifford Brooke, "Sex(haustion) Sells: Marketing in a Saturated Mediascape," in *Sex in Advertising: Perspectives on the Erotic Appeal*, ed. Tom Reicher and Jacqueline Lambiase (Mahwah, NJ: Lawrence Erlbaum Associates, Inc., 2003): 136; Benjamin Svetkey, "Jenny on the Spot," *Entertainment*, October 10, 1997.

7. Jenny McCarthy and Neal Karlen, *Jen-X: Jenny McCarthy's Open Book* (New York: Harpercollins, 1997); Amazon.com, "Review of *Jen-X*," www.amazon.com/Jen-X-Jenny-McCarthys-Open-Book/dp/0060392339/ref=sr_1_1?ie=UTF8&s=books&qid=1279890171&sr=8-1 (accessed July 23, 2010); Jenny McCarthy, *Belly Laughs: The Naked Truth about Pregnancy and Childbirth* (New York: De Capo Books, 2004); McCarthy, *Baby Laughs: The Naked Truth about the First Year of Motherhood* (New York: Dutton Adult, 2005); Tori Spelling, *sTORI Telling* (New York: Simon Spotlight, 2008); Spelling, *Mommywood* (New York: Simon Spotlight, 2009).

8. Jenny McCarthy, *Life Laughs: The Naked Truth About Motherhood, Marriage, and Moving On* (New York: Dutton, 2006), 1.

9. Jenny McCarthy, *Louder Than Words: A Mother's Journey in Healing Autism* (New York: Dutton, 2007), 1–9, 11.

10. Barbara Sibbald, "It's Wise to Immunize, Regardless of What the Web Says," *Journal of the Canadian Medical Association* 161 (199): 736; Jennifer Keelan, Vera Pavri-Garcia, George Tomilson, and Kumanan Wilson, "Research Letter: YouTube as a Source of Information on Immunization; A Content Analysis," *Journal of the American Medical Association* 298 (2007): 2482–88; Laeth Nasir, "Reconnoitering the Anti-vaccination Web Sites: News from the Front," *Journal of Family Practice* 49 (2000): 731–33; Robert M. Wolfe, Lisa K. Sharp, and Martin S. Lipsky, "Content and Design Attributes of Anti-vaccination Web Sites," *Journal of the American Medical Association* 287 (2002): 3245–48; P. Davies, S. Chapman, and J. Leask, "Anti-vaccination Activists on the World Wide Web," *Archives of Disease in Childhood* 87 (2002): 22–25; Richard K. Zimmerman, Robert M. Wolfe, Dwight E. Fox, Jake R. Fox, Mary Patricia Nowalk, Judith A. Troy, and Lisa K. Sharp, "Vaccine Criticism on the World Wide Web," *Journal of Medical Internet Research* 7 (2005): e17.

11. McCarthy, *Louder Than Words*, 47, 77.

12. Pilar Guzmán, "Jenny McCarthy," *Cookie,* September 2009; McCarthy, *Louder Than Words*, 83.

13. Lisa S. Lewis, *Special Diets for Special Kids: Understanding and Implementing a Gluten and Casein Free Diet to Aid in the Treatment of Autism and Related Developmental Disorders* (Arlington, TX: Future Horizons, Inc., 1998), 35.

14. McCarthy, *Louder Than Words*, 105, 107.

15. E. Ernst, "Chelation Therapy for Coronary Heart Disease: An Overview of All Clinical Investigations," *American Heart Journal* 140 (2000): 139–41; Merril L. Knudtson, George Wyse, P. Diane Galbraith, Rolling Brant, Kathy Hildebrand, Diana Paterson, Deborah Richardson, Connie Burkart, and Ellen Burgess, "Chelation Therapy for Ischemic Heart Disease: A Randomized Controlled Trial," *Journal of the American Medical Association* 287 (2002): 481–86; Yashwant Shinha, Natalie Silove, and Katrina Williams, "Chelation Therapy and Autism," *British Medical Journal* 333 (2006): 756; Daniel B. Rubin, "Letter to the Editor: Fanning the Vaccine-Autism Link," *Neurology Today* 8 (2008): 3; Karl Taro Greenfeld, "The Autism Debate: Who's Afraid of Jenny McCarthy?" *Time,* February 25, 2010.

16. Cris Italia, "Jenny and Jim Rally Thousands," *Spectrum* (August/September 2008).

17. Ibid.; Jeffrey Kluger, "Jenny McCarthy on Autism and Vaccines," *Time,* April 1, 2009.

18. Jenny McCarthy, *Mother Warriors* (New York: Dutton, 2008); Jenny McCarthy and Jerry Kartzinel, *Healing and Preventing Autism: A Complete Guide* (New York: Dutton, 2009), 278.

19. "Jenny McCarthy and Holly Robinson Peete—Their Fight to Save Their Autistic Sons," *The Oprah Winfrey Show,* September 18, 2007; Message Boards, "Oprah.com Community: Jenny McCarthy and Holly Robinson Peete," www.oprah.com/community/threat/1542 (accessed April 15, 2008).

20. Arthur Allen, "Say It Ain't So, O: Why is Oprah Winfrey Promoting Vaccine Skeptic Jenny McCarthy?" *Slate,* May 6, 2009.

21. Greenfeld, "The Autism Debate."

22. Paul A. Offit and Louis Bell, *Vaccines: What You Should Know* (Hoboken: John Wiley, 2003); Offit, *The Cutter Incident: How America's First Polio Vaccine Led to Today's Growing Vaccine Crisis* (New Haven: Yale, 2005); Offit, *Vaccinated: One*

Man's Quest to Defeat the World's Deadliest Diseases (New York: Smithsonian Books, 2007); Offit, *Autism's False Prophets: Bad Science, Risky Medicine, and the Search for a Cure* (New York: Columbia University Press, 2008).

23. "Pertussis and Keri Russell," www.pkids.org/dis_pert_keri-russell-bio.php (accessed July 27, 2010); Jonann Brady, "Jennifer Lopez Getting Her Work Mojo Back: Lopez Talks about Marc, Twins, Career, and Raising Whooping Cough Awareness," *Good Morning America*, April 22, 2009; E. J. Mundell, "Jennifer Garner Puts Flu Shot in the Spotlight: Actress and New Mom Calls Vaccines 'Family Priority' This Season," *U.S. News and World Report*, July 26, 2010; Elizabeth Snead, "Charlie Sheen Tells Denise Richards: Don't Stick My Kids!" *The Dishrag*, http://blog.zap2it.com/thedishrag/2008/06/charlie-sheen-t.html (accessed July 27, 2010).

24. Jennifer Tung, "Amanda Peet," *Cookie*, August 2008.

25. cookiemag.com>forms>hot topics, "Amanda Peet/Vaccines," *Cookie*, http://boards.cookiemag.com/thread.jspa?threadID=849&tstart=0 (accessed July 14, 2009); Amanda Peet, "Amanda Peet's Response," *Cookie*, www.cookiemag.com/entertainment/2008/07/peet_apology.

26. "Get Up To Speed on the Vaccine Debate," *Cookie*, www.cookiemag.com/entertainment/2008/07/vaccine_experts?printable=true&currentPage=all (accessed July 14, 2009).

27. Paul Costello and Rosanne Spector, "Peet's Passion: The Medical Education of Amanda Peet," *Stanford Medical Magazine* (Spring 2009); Dan Childs, "X-Files Actress on Vaccines: Ignore the Stars," *ABC News*, http://abcnews.go.com/print?=5483159.

28. Dan Childs, "X-Files Actress on Vaccines: Ignore the Stars," *ABC News*, http://abcnews.go.com/print?=5483159.

29. Andrew Zoltan, "*Jacobson* Revisited: Mandatory Polio Vaccination as an Unconstitutional Condition," *George Mason Law Review* 735 (2004–6): 744. Supreme Court of the United States, *Jacobson v. Commonwealth of Massachusetts*, 197 U.S. 11 (1905).

30. Wendy K. Mariner, George J. Annas, and Leonard H. Glantz, "*Jacobson v. Massachusetts*: It's Not Your Great-Great-Grandfather's Public Health Law," *American Journal of Public Health* 95 (2005).

31. Colgrove and Bayer, "Manifold Restraints: Liberty, Public Health, and the Legacy of *Jacobson v. Massachusetts*," *American Journal of Public Health* 4 (2005): 571.

32. Jacob Heller, *The Vaccine Narrative* (Nashville: Vanderbilt University Press 2008); "Toward a Twenty-First-Century *Jacobson v. Massachusetts*," *Harvard Law Review* 121 (2008): 1820–41.

33. Office of the United Nations High Commissioner for Human Rights and the Joint United Nations Programme on HIV/AIDS, *HIV/AIDS and Human Rights: International Guidelines* (New York: United Nations, 1998); Colgrove and Bayer, "Manifold Restraints," 574–75; George J. Annas, "Blinded by Bioterrorism: Public Health and Liberty in the 21st Century," *Health Matrix* 13 (2003): 33–70.

34. Warren E. Leary, "Barriers to Immunization Peril Children, Experts Say," *New York Times*, April 24, 1994; Robert Pear, "The Health Care Debate: Immunizations," *New York Times*, August 23, 1994; Deborah Franklin, "To Vaccinate or Not? Sorting Out the Confusion Over Meningitis Shots," *New York Times*, June 28, 2005.

35. Gina Kolata, "A Nation Challenged: Vaccinations," *New York Times,* March 20, 2002; Personal Correspondence with Michael Nelson, August 10, 2010.

CHAPTER 6: Getting to the Source of Anxiety

1. Donald G. McNeil Jr., "Book Is Rallying Resistance to the Anti-vaccine Crusade," *New York Times,* January 12, 2009.

2. MedlinePlus Medical Encyclopedia, "Well Child Visits," www.nlm.nih.gov /medlineplus/ency/article/001928.htm (accessed July 28, 2010).

3. For an excellent exploration of this topic, see Carl Elliott, *Better Than Well: American Medicine Meets the American Dream* (New York: W. W. Norton & Co., 2003).

4. Janeen Interlandi and Raina Kelley, "What Addicts Need," *Newsweek,* March 3, 2008, 37–42; Ronald Kotulak, "Anti-Addiction Vaccines Raise Ethics Questions," *The Lansing State Journal,* October 1, 2006, 11A; David Brown, "Vaccine Against Heroin Works—At Least in Rats," *Washington Post,* July 25, 2011; Jeneen Interlandi, "Are Vaccines the Answer to Addiction?" *Newsweek,* January 14, 2008, 17; Barbara Fox, "Development of a Therapeutic Vaccine for the Treatment of Cocaine Addiction," *Drug and Alcohol Dependence* 48 (1997): 153–58; "New Type of Vaccine against Nicotine Addiction Developed by TSRI Scientists," *ScienceDaily,* May 21, 2003, www .sciencedaily.com/releases/2003/05/030521092701.htm (accessed December 12, 2007); Michael M. Meijler, Masayuki Matsushita, Laurence J. Altobell III, Peter Wirsching, and Kim D. Janda, "A New Strategy for Improving Nicotine Vaccines Using Conformationally Constrained Haptens," *Journal of the American Chemical Society* 125 (2003): 7164–65; Nicole Garbarini, "Cocaine Vaccine," *Scientific American,* December 2004; Todd Ackerman, "Houston Scientists See Hope in Cocaine Vaccine," *Houston Chronicle,* January 1, 2008; S. Goodchild and S. Bloomfield, "Children to Get Jabs against Drug Addiction: Ministers Consider Vaccination Scheme in Heroine, Cocaine, and Nicotine," *Independent on Sunday,* July 25, 2004; Peter J. Cohen, "Prevention and Treatment of Cocaine Abuse: Ethical and Legal Considerations," *Drug and Alcohol Dependence* 47 (1997): 167–74; Alexis Osburn, "Immunizing Against Addiction: The Argument for Incorporating Emerging Anti-addiction Vaccines into Existing Compulsory Immunization Statues," *Cleveland State Law Review* 56 (2008): 159–88.

5. Stanley A. Plotkin, "Vaccines: Past, Present and Future," *Nature Medicine* 11 (2005): S5. According to the CDC, the twenty-seven currently vaccine-preventable diseases are anthrax, cervical cancer, diphtheria, hepatitis A and B, *Haemophilus influenzae* type b, human papillomavirus, influenza, Japanese encephalitis, Lyme disease, measles, meningococcal, monkeypox, mumps, pertussis, poliomyelitis, rabies, rotavirus, rubella, shingles, smallpox, tetanus, tuberculosis, typhoid fever, varicella, and yellow fever. Centers for Disease Control and Prevention, "Vaccines: VPD-VAC/ VPD menu page," www.cdc.gov/vaccines/vpd-vac/default.htm (accessed. December 18, 2008); U.S. National Institutes of Health, "Search of: vaccine | Open Studies— List Results—ClinicalTrials.gov," http://clinicaltrials.gov/ct2/results?term=vaccine& recr=Open&rslt=&type=&cond=&intr=&spons=&id=&state1=&cntry1=&state2=& cntry2=&state3=&cntry3=&locn=&rcv_s=&rcv_e=&lup_s=&lup_e= (accessed, January 2, 2009).

6. Francis Fukuyama, *Our Posthuman Future: Consequences of the Biotechnology Revolution* (New York: Picador, 2002), 7.

7. Alina Salganicof, Usha R. Ranji, and Roerta Wyn, *Women and Health Care: A National Survey; Key Findings from the Kaiser Women's Health Survey* (Washington, DC: Henry J. Kaiser Family Foundation, 2005), vii.

8. For discussions of the differences between men and women on the subject of health care, see Marta Gil-Lacruz and Ana I. Gil-Lacruz, "Health Perception and Health Care Access: Sex Differences in Behaviors and Attitudes," *American Journal of Economics and Sociology* 69 (2010): 783–801; Naranjana Mani, "Gender Differences in Risk Perceptions and Health Beliefs Related to Tobacco Use," presented at the American Public Health Association Annual Meeting, November 4–8, 2006; D. G. Safran, W. H. Rogers, A. R. Tarlov, C. A. McHorney, and J. E. Ware Jr., "Gender Differences in Medical Treatment: The Case of Physician-Prescribed Restrictions," *Social Science and Medicine* 45 (1997): 711–22; Tyrone F. Borders, Ke Tom Zu, James Heavner, and Gina Kruse, "Patient Involvement in Medical Decision-making among Elder: Physician or Patient-Driven?" *BMC Health Services Research* 5 (2005).

9. Kerry Howley, "Until Cryonics Do Us Part," *New York Times,* July 5, 2010; Ari Schulman, "Are 'Hostile Wives' Too Cool Toward Science?" *The New Atlantic Blogs,* July 26, 2010.

10. U.S. Food and Drug Administration, Center for Biologics Evaluation and Research, "How Does FDA Evaluate Vaccines to Make Sure They Are Safe?" www.hhs.gov/fda/faq/vaccines/1856.html (July 26, 2010); Centers for Disease Control and Prevention, "CDC—Testing and Monitoring—Vaccine Safety," www.cdc.gov/vaccinesafety/Vaccine_Monitoring/Index.html (accessed July 27, 2010).

11. Vaccine Adverse Event Reporting System, "About the VAERS Program," http://vaers.hhs.gov/about/index (accessed July 27, 2010); M. Miles Braun, "Vaccine Adverse Event Reporting System (VAERS): Usefulness and Limitations," www.vaccinesafety.edu/VAERS.htm (accessed July 26, 2010).

12. Vaccine Adverse Event Reporting System, "VAERS Data," http://vaers.hhs.gov/data/index (accessed July 26, 2010); S. Rosenthal S and R. Chen, "The Reporting Sensitivities of Two Passive Surveillance Systems for Vaccine Adverse Events," *American Journal of Public Health* 85 (1995): 1706–9; J. C. P. Weber, "Epidemiology of Adverse Reactions to Non-steroidal Anti-inflammatory Drugs," *Advances in Inflammation Research* 6 (1984): 1–7; Paul A. Offit, *Autism's False Prophets: Bad Science, Risky Medicine, and the Search for a Cure* (New York: Columbia University Press, 2008), 138. Offit cited Michael Goodman, "Vaccine Adverse Event Reporting System Reporting Source: A Possible Source of Bias in Longitudinal Studies," *Pediatrics* 117 (2006): 387–90.

13. Michele Gillen, "HPV Scientist Speaks Out," WFOR-TV, http://cbs4.com/iteam/Gardisil.Girls.Vaccine.2.718592.html (accessed July 26, 2010).

14. Robert W. Sears, *The Vaccine Book: Making the Right Choice for Your Child* (New York: Little, Brown and Co., 2007), 222–23; Paul A. Offit and Charlotte A. Moser, "The Problem with Dr. Bob's Alternative Vaccine Schedule," *Pediatrics* 123 (2009): 164–69. For an example of the ways in which the dispute between Offit and Sears has been described, see Brian P. Bowman, "eLetters for Offit and Moster, 'Front Line' Response to the Vaccine Book," *Pediatrics* (December 20, 2008), http://pediatrics.aappublications.org/cgi/eletters/123/1/e164 (accessed July 26, 2010); Joseph T. Malak,

"eLetters for Offit and Moster, Backfire," *Pediatrics* (December 31, 2008), http://pedi atrics.aappublications.org/cgi/eletters/123/1/e164 (accessed July 26, 2010); Jon S. Poling, "eLetters for Offit and Moster, View from the Other Side and 'Scientific Proofs,'" *Pediatrics* (January 2, 2009), http://pediatrics.aappublications.org/cgi/eletters/123/1 /e164 (accessed July 26, 2010); Steven Novella, "Paul Offit Takes on Robert Sears," *Science-Based Medicine: Exploring Issues and Controversies in the Relationship between Science and Medicine* (January 7, 2009), www.sciencebasedmedicine.org /?p=333 (accessed July 26, 2010); Deborah Kotz, "Flexible Approach to Vaccinations Comes Under Fire," *U.S. News and World Report*, December 29, 2008; "Offit vs. Sears—Anti-Vaccine Media Bias," *Parenting Solved: Compelling Commentary on Children's Health* (January 2, 2009), http://parentingsolved.typepad.com/parenting _solved/2009/01/offit-vs-sears-anti-vaccine.html (accessed July 26, 2010).

15. Sarah Abruzzese, "Maryland Parents Told to Have Children Immunized," *New York Times*, November 18, 2007; "Parents Ordered to Court of Kids' Shots," *New York Times*, November 19, 2007; Alexandra Stewart, "Challenging Personal Belief Immunization Exemptions: Considering Legal Responses," *Michigan Law Review* 107 (2009): 105–9; James Colgrove and Ronald Bayer, "Manifold Restraints: Liberty, Public Health, and the Legacy of *Jacobson v. Massachusetts*," *American Journal of Public Health* 4 (2005): 571.

16. Deborah L. Shelton, "Some Pediatricians Taking Stand for Vaccine Program," *Chicago Tribune*, July 6, 2011; Douglas S. Diekema, "Responding to Parental Refusals of Immunization of Children," *Pediatrics* 115, no. 5 (2005).

17. Margaret S. Coleman, Megan C. Lindley, John Ekong, and Lance Rodewald, "Net Financial Gain or Loss from Vaccination in Pediatric Medical Practices," *Pediatrics* 124 (2009): S472–91.

18. Colman, et al., "Net Financial Gain or Loss from Vaccination," S477. Brian P. Bowman, "eLetters for Offit and Moster, 'Front Line' Response to the Vaccine Book," *Pediatrics* (December 20, 2008), http://pediatrics.aappublications.org/cgi/eletters/123 /1/e164 (accessed July 26, 2010).

INDEX

DATE DUE